Mental Health Issues in Lesbian, Gay, Bisexual, and Transgender Communities

Review of Psychiatry Series

John M. Oldham, M.D., M.S.
Michelle B. Riba, M.D., M.S.
Series Editors

Mental Health Issues in Lesbian, Gay, Bisexual, and Transgender Communities

EDITED BY

Billy E. Jones, M.D., M.S.

Marjorie J. Hill, Ph.D.

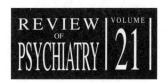

REVIEW OF PSYCHIATRY VOLUME 21

No. 4

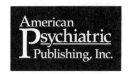

American Psychiatric Publishing, Inc.

Washington, DC
London, England

Note: The authors have worked to ensure that all information in this book concerning drug dosages, schedules, and routes of administration is accurate as of the time of publication and consistent with standards set by the U.S. Food and Drug Administration and the general medical community. As medical research and practice advance, however, therapeutic standards may change. For this reason and because human and mechanical errors sometimes occur, we recommend that readers follow the advice of a physician who is directly involved in their care or the care of a member of their family. A product's current package insert should be consulted for full prescribing and safety information.

Books published by American Psychiatric Publishing, Inc., represent the views and opinions of the individual authors and do not necessarily represent the policies and opinions of APPI or the American Psychiatric Association.

American Psychiatric Publishing, Inc.
1400 K Street, NW
Washington, DC 20005
www.appi.org

The correct citation for this book is

Jones BE, Hill MJ (editors): *Mental Health Issues in Lesbian, Gay, Bisexual, and Transgender Communities* (Review of Psychiatry Series, Volume 21, Number 4; Oldham JM and Riba MB, series editors). Washington, DC, American Psychiatric Publishing, 2002

Library of Congress Cataloging-in-Publication Data
Mental health issues in lesbian, gay, bisexual, and transgender communities / edited by Billy E. Jones, Marjorie J. Hill.
     p. ; cm. — (Review of psychiatry series ; v. 21, no. 4)
  Includes bibliographical references and index.
  ISBN 1-58562-069-6 (alk. paper)
    1. Gays—Mental health. 2. Bisexuals—Mental health. 3. Transsexuals—Mental health. I. Jones, Billy E., 1938–   II. Hill, Marjorie J. III. Review of psychiatry series ; v. 21, 4
  RC451.4.G39 M45 2002
  362.2′086′64—dc21

                2002022755

British Library Cataloguing in Publication Data
A CIP record is available from the British Library.

To Lewis, my partner of 35 years,
with much love
Billy

Contents

Chapter 3
Offering Psychiatric Opinion in Legal Proceedings
When Lesbian or Gay Sexual Orientation Is an Issue 37
Richard G. Dudley Jr., M.D.

Chapter 4
Sexual Conversion ("Reparative") Therapies:
History and Update 71
Jack Drescher, M.D.

Chapter 5

**Transgender Mental Health: The Intersection of
Race, Sexual Orientation, and Gender Identity**
Donald E. Tarver II, M.D.

Contributors

Jeffrey S. Akman, M.D.
The Leon M. Yochelson Professor and Interim Chair, Department of Psychiatry and Behavioral Sciences, George Washington University, Washington, D.C.

Jack Drescher, M.D.
Chair, American Psychiatric Association Committee on Gay, Lesbian and Bisexual Issues; Training and Supervising Analyst, William Alanson White Psychoanalytic Institute, New York City; Clinical Assistant Professor of Psychiatry, State University of New York—Brooklyn

Richard G. Dudley Jr., M.D.
Private Practice, New York, New York

Barry Fisher, M.D.
Chief Resident, Department of Psychiatry and Behavioral Sciences, George Washington University, Washington, D.C.

Marjorie J. Hill, Ph.D.
Acting Assistant Commissioner for HIV Services, New York City Department of Health; Board Member, National Gay and Lesbian Task Force; Member, New York Association of Black Psychologists

Billy E. Jones, M.D., M.S.
Chief Consultant, B. Jones Consulting Service; Clinical Professor of Psychiatry and Behavioral Sciences, New York Medical College, New York, New York

Douglas C. Kimmel, Ph.D.
Professor Emeritus, Department of Psychology, City College, City University of New York

John M. Oldham, M.D., M.S.
Dollard Professor and Acting Chairman, Department of Psychiatry, Columbia University College of Physicians and Surgeons, New York, New York

Michelle B. Riba, M.D., M.S.
Associate Chair for Education and Academic Affairs, Department of Psychiatry, University of Michigan Medical School, Ann Arbor, Michigan

Donald E. Tarver II, M.D.
Clinical Lecturer, University of California, San Francisco

Introduction to the Review of Psychiatry Series

John M. Oldham, M.D., M.S.
Michelle B. Riba, M.D., M.S., Series Editors

2002 REVIEW OF PSYCHIATRY SERIES TITLES

- *Cutting-Edge Medicine: What Psychiatrists Need to Know*
  EDITED BY NADA L. STOTLAND, M.D., M.P.H.
- *The Many Faces of Depression in Children and Adolescents*
  EDITED BY DAVID SHAFFER, F.R.C.P.(LOND), F.R.C.PSYCH.(LOND),
  AND BRUCE D. WASLICK, M.D.
- *Emergency Psychiatry*
  EDITED BY MICHAEL H. ALLEN, M.D.
- *Mental Health Issues in Lesbian, Gay, Bisexual, and Transgender Communities*
  EDITED BY BILLY E. JONES, M.D., M.S., AND MARJORIE J. HILL, PH.D.

There is a growing literature describing the stress–vulnerability model of illness, a model applicable to many, if not most, psychiatric disorders and to physical illness as well. Vulnerability comes in a number of forms. Genetic predisposition to specific conditions may arise as a result of spontaneous mutations, or it may be transmitted intergenerationally in family pedigrees. Secondary types of vulnerability may involve susceptibility to disease caused by the weakened resistance that accompanies malnutrition, immunocompromised states, and other conditions. In most of these models of illness, vulnerability consists of a necessary but not sufficient precondition; if specific stresses are avoided, or if they are encountered but offset by adequate protective factors, the disease does not manifest itself and the vulnerability may never be recognized. Conversely, there is increasing recognition of the role of stress as a precipitant of frank illness in vulnerable individuals and of the complex and subtle interactions among the environment, emotions, and neurodevelopmental, metabolic, and physiological processes.

In this country, the years 2001 and 2002 contained stress of unprecedented proportions, with the terrorist attacks on September 11 and the events that followed that terrible day. Although the contents of Volume 21 of the Review of Psychiatry were well established by that date and much of the text had already been written, we could not introduce this volume without thinking about the relevance of this unanticipated, widespread stress to the topics already planned.

Certainly, major depression is one of the prime candidates among the disorders in vulnerable populations that can be precipitated by stress. The information presented in *The Many Faces of Depression in Children and Adolescents*, edited by David Shaffer and Bruce D. Waslick, is, then, timely indeed. Already identified as a growing problem in youth—all too often accompanied by suicidal behavior—depression in children and adolescents is especially important to identify as early as possible. School-based screening services need to be widespread in order to facilitate both prevention of the disorder in those at risk and referral for effective treatment for those already experiencing symptomatic depression. Both psychotherapy and pharmacotherapy are well established as effective treatments for this condition, making recognition of its presence even more important. In New York alone, thousands of children lost at least one parent in the World Trade Center disaster, a catastrophic event precipitating not just grief but also major depression in the children and adolescents at risk.

We now know that stress, and depression itself, affect not just the brain but the body as well. New information about this brain–body axis is provided in *Cutting-Edge Medicine: What Psychiatrists Need to Know*, edited by Nada L. Stotland. Depression as an independent risk factor for cardiac death is one of the new findings reviewed in the chapter on the mind and the heart, as we understand more about the interactions among emotions, behavior, and cardiovascular functioning. Similarly, stress and mood are primary players in the homeostasis, or lack of it, of other body systems, such as the menstrual cycle and gastrointestinal functioning, also reviewed in this book. Finally, the massive increase in organ transplantation, in which medical advances have made it possible to neutralize the body's own immune responses against foreign tissue, represents a new frontier in which emotional stability is critical in donor and recipient.

Increasingly, medicine's front door is the hospital emergency service. Not just a place where triage occurs, though that remains an important and challenging function, the psychiatric emergency service needs to have expert clinicians who can perform careful assessments and initiate treatment. The latest thinking by psychiatrists experienced in emergency work is presented in *Emergency Psychiatry*, edited by Michael H. Allen. Certainly, psychiatric emergency services serve as one of the most critical components of the response network that needs to be in place to deal with a disaster such as the September 2001 attack and the bioterrorism events that followed.

Perhaps less obviously linked to those September events, *Mental Health Issues in Lesbian, Gay, Bisexual, and Transgender Communities*, edited by Billy E. Jones and Marjorie J. Hill, which reviews current thinking about gay, lesbian, bisexual, and transgender issues, reflects our changing world in other ways. A continuing process is necessary as we rethink our assumptions and challenge and question any prejudice or bias that may have infiltrated our thinking or may have been embedded in our traditional concepts. In this book, traditional notions are contrasted with newer thinking about gender role and sexual orientation, considering these issues from youth to old age, as we continue to try to differentiate the wide range of human diversity from what we classify as illness.

We believe that the topics covered in Volume 21 are timely and represent a selection of important updates for the practicing clinician. Next year, this tradition will continue, with books on trauma and disaster response and management, edited by Robert J. Ursano and Ann E. Norwood; on molecular neurobiology for the clinician, edited by Dennis S. Charney; on geriatric psychiatry, edited by Alan M. Mellow; and on standardized assessment for the clinician, edited by Michael B. First.

Preface

Billy E. Jones, M.D., M.S.
Marjorie J. Hill, Ph.D.

$\mathbf{W}$e have witnessed an astonishing growth in the literature and study of homosexuality over the past few decades (Cabaj and Stein 1996). Experts such as Hooker, Duberman, Isay, and Silverstein, to name only a few, have helped to research, explore, and explain the modern concept of a gay and lesbian identity and have presented and discussed many associated mental health issues (Duberman 1991, 1993; Hooker 1957; Isay 1996, 1989; Silverstein 1991). Mental heath professionals, students, and others now have a field of study from which to gain knowledge, data, concepts, and education about the members of lesbian, gay, bisexual, and transgender communities.

But this field of study is young, and as in any young field there is much to learn. There are still many issues affecting the mental health of the members of lesbian, gay, bisexual, and transgender communities that have not been discussed or sufficiently presented. This volume presents some of these issues with the hope that an understanding of these issues will help professionals better differentiate health from pathology and more accurately evaluate and successfully treat lesbian, gay, bisexual, and transgender persons.

This topic is not only important but also surprisingly timely. Over the last couple of years in our country the media have finally begun to include healthy images of gay men and lesbians in the cast of characters in television shows, movies, books, and other presentations for the public. While the country is growing accustomed to seeing openly gay men, lesbians, and bisexuals with more frequency, and some walls of prejudice are definitely crumbling, there remains a tremendous need for the populace at large to better understand the members of the lesbian, gay, bisexual, and transgender communities and the issues affecting them. The mental health community plays an important role in helping to more fully explain the issues relevant to these communities to the larger society and enhancing their assimilation into the mainstream.

While the words *lesbian, gay, bisexual,* and *transgender* have come to be referred to with one phrase—the LGBT community—used to symbolize a group of individuals who have a different sexual lifestyle than the majority heterosexual individuals in our society, there are in fact four communities. Each community is different—not only from the heterosexual community but from each other—and in some ways unique. In addition, each community is diverse. What this means is that what seems generally to be the case in the lesbian community may not be the case in the gay men's community. What is generally the case with white gay men may not be the case with African American gay men. Even with the differences among communities and the diversity within each community, there are some common mental health issues. In discussing these issues in this book, the authors attempt to address the similarities and differences, as well as to acknowledge the diversity, in lesbian, gay, bisexual, and transgender communities.

All the talented, professional contributors to this book have done an extraordinary job of addressing the important issues in their chapters. They provide the reader with a thorough review of the subject matter, provide us with the current state of knowledge, introduce new information, and propose additional avenues of inquiry. Some of the issues and topics presented in this book, such as lesbian, gay, bisexual, and transgender youth and sexual conversion therapy, have an existing body of knowledge to which the current authors are adding. Other of the topics presented—such as aging in the lesbian, gay, bisexual, and transgender community; offering psychiatric opinion in legal proceedings in which sexual orientation is an issue; and transgender mental health—have very little, if anything, written about them. In the latter cases, the authors are helping to initiate a knowledge base.

In Chapter 1, Drs. Fisher and Akman present a thorough review of the mental health literature on sexual minority youth.

They discuss normal adolescent development and the extra challenges imposed by the development of a sexual identity that is different from that of most of their peers. The lack of lesbian, gay, bisexual, and transgender role models is one of the many issues pointed out that makes successful development more difficult. Other mental health issues of sexual minority youth are discussed.

The infrequently addressed subject of aging and sexual orientation presents a historical background of the current cohorts of older lesbian, bisexual, and gay adults. In Chapter 2, Dr. Kimmel discusses theoretical models and empirical data on aging as a stigmatized sexual minority. The similarities and differences of aging between the sexual minority communities and the heterosexual community, including ageism and heterosexism, are discussed. Special issues in working with aging ethnic minority gay men, lesbians, and bisexual persons are also stressed.

Legal proceedings involving individuals with same-sex orientation often require psychiatrists to offer a psychiatric opinion. In Chapter 3, Dr. Dudley discusses many of the issues, false assumptions, and lack of knowledge involved when lesbians and gay men are involved in child custody or visitation proceedings, workplace harassment and other discrimination cases, criminal law and same-sex domestic violence cases, and immigration and asylum cases. This chapter presents issues rarely, if ever, discussed.

In Chapter 4, on sexual conversion ("reparative") therapies, Dr. Drescher writes about the three types of etiological theories on homosexuality presented in the scientific literature and provides a historical overview of clinical attitudes toward homosexuality to the present. He reports on adverse side effects of sexual conversion treatments and raises important clinical and ethical concerns about these therapies.

Very little has been written about mental health issues in the transgender community. Dr. Tarver, in Chapter 5, presents the argument that the increased visibility of successfully functioning transgender persons confronts and undermines the rationale for a specific designation of diagnoses of transvestism, transsexualism, or gender identity disorder. The author explains that just as the concepts of psychiatric disease and remedy are no longer based on racial or homosexual identity, they should not be based on gender identity.

Undoubtedly, there is much to be added to the growing body of knowledge of mental health issues in the lesbian, gay, bisexual, and transgender communities. We hope this book is informative, contributes to your knowledge, and enhances your skills.

References

Cabaj RP, Stein TS (eds): Textbook of Homosexuality and Mental Health. Washington, DC, American Psychiatric Press, 1996

Duberman MB: Cures: A Gay Man's Odyssey. New York, Dutton, 1991

Duberman MB: Stonewall. New York, Plume, 1993

Hooker E: The adjustment of the male overt homosexual. Journal of Projective Techniques 21:18–31, 1957

Isay R: Being Homosexual. New York, Farrar, Straus & Giroux, 1989

Isay R: Becoming Gay: The Journey to Self-Acceptance. New York, Pantheon, 1996

Silverstein C (ed): Gays, Lesbians, and Their Therapists: Studies in Psychotherapy. New York, WW Norton, 1991

Chapter 1

Normal Development in Sexual Minority Youth

Barry Fisher, M.D.
Jeffrey S. Akman, M.D.

In this chapter, we discuss normal, healthy sexual development in sexual minority youth. In the process, we address issues of identity development and the coming-out process, including school experiences (including issues of harassment and violence), parental acceptance and family relationships, and availability and use of social supports like the Gay/Straight Alliances found at some schools. Dating and sexual activity are discussed, as is the impact of ethnic and cultural diversity. We also examine the unique developmental issues for bisexual and transgender youth. In the process, we review the most widely accepted theories on sexual minority development and discuss the most recent data from studies of sexual minority youth.

The term *sexual minority* is used whenever possible to include four distinct groups: gay male, lesbian, bisexual, and transgender individuals. In some ways using an umbrella term like *sexual minority youth* is difficult and, at times, unwieldy. We recognize that the development of lesbians differs from that of gay males, which differs even further from the development of bisexual or transgender persons. However, using this term has advantages in that the discussion is not limited to gay and lesbian issues. Where possible, we make distinctions among the four groups. When prior studies are cited, we provide a context for which group was actually studied.

Sexual Minority Identity Development

All adolescents experience the same developmental tasks, which involve physical, cognitive, social, and emotional growth. Most of these tasks have little or nothing to do with sexual identity development. However, sexual minority youth face extra challenges that those in the majority do not: experiencing the development of a sexual identity different from most, if not all, of those around them and integrating that identity into a healthy, overall view of themselves as worthwhile individuals (Rotheram-Borus and Fernandez 1995).

Models of Identity Development

In 1979 Vivienne Cass set out a six-stage model of identity formation: confusion, comparison, tolerance, acceptance, pride, and synthesis (Cass 1979). Cass's system is based on levels of increasing self-understanding. The theory attempts to explain how self-awareness grows in a complex interaction between self-reflection and assimilation of the culture in which one lives. The model is purposefully flexible and allows movement back and forth between stages as sexual identity develops. Further, the theory is designed to encompass anyone who develops a sexual identity outside the societal norm of heterosexuality. As Cass (1996, p. 233) noted, "the psychological process of confronting personal information that relates to membership in a stigmatized social category is considered a generic one. Informal adaptations of the model have already been made to bisexual and cross-dressing individuals."

Cass's model focuses on the thoughts and feelings that someone might have in a given stage so that effective therapeutic interventions can be designed for each stage of self-awareness. In particular, Cass focuses on the defense mechanisms an individual might use during any given stage. For example, denial is a primary defense in stage 1, and rationalization is a primary defense in stage 2. In stage 3, one may adopt an asexual persona or practice covert homosexual behavior. In stage 4, an individual might consciously split his or her identity and act heterosexual in public while acknowledging a bisexual or homosexual identity in private. In stages 3 and 4, denial, suppression, avoidance, reaction formation, and other midlevel defenses may be utilized. Experiencing feelings of pride and anger, publicly pronouncing one's sexual identity, and viewing the world with an "us vs. them" mentality may be used in stage 5. Stage 6 is devoted to identity integration and maturity. Sexual identity is seen as only a part of one's overall identity and not the defining characteristic. Individuals develop a sense of mastery and control of their lives and outwardly display more independence and self-confidence.

In 1982, Coleman described five developmental stages: pre–coming out, coming out, exploration, first relationships, and identity integration (see Beaty 1999). This theory focuses primarily on self-awareness in the first two stages and on developmental tasks in the last three. In the pre–coming-out stage, individuals see themselves as different from others, and they acknowledge homosexual feelings in the coming-out stage. In the third stage, three developmental tasks are stressed: they acquire interpersonal skills for meeting others like them, develop a sense of personal attractiveness, and learn that healthy self-esteem is not gained through sexual activity alone. Individuals learn same-sex relationship skills in the fourth stage. The last stage is marked by integrating public and private images into one identity.

In 1979, Troiden theorized four age-specific developmental stages. The first, *sensitization*, occurs before puberty and is described as a vague awareness that one is somehow different from same-sex peers. The second, *identity confusion*, generally occurs in adolescence and involves inner turmoil that one might be gay. The third, *identity assumption*, occurs in late adolescence or early adulthood as the individual begins to explore sexuality and gay subculture. The fourth, *commitment*, occurs when a gay identity is perceived as necessary for optimal functioning (Zera 1992).

The three models described above try to explain sexual minority identity development in the context of a culture that stigmatizes sexual minorities. They imply that development occurs over an extended period of time and involves disclosure to others at some point during the developmental process.

Self-Identity Issues

Many studies suggest that sexual minorities, particularly gay men, experience an awareness that they are "different" as early as age 4 (Isay 1987, 1989, 1991; Siegel and Lowe 1994; Telljohann and Price 1993).

Gay adolescents generally begin to question their sexual orientation between the ages of 12 and 14. Because the capacity for abstract thought has developed by this period, adolescents are able to analyze their responses to others and place those responses and the feelings that accompany them into a larger context (Zera 1992). They may become more aware of behavior that is considered gender atypical, having sexual or emotional fantasies involving a same-gender friend, or feeling aroused when seeing or touching someone of the same sex. Individuals will also realize that those feelings are likely to be viewed negatively by their society. Many may begin to fear humiliation or even physical violence if others discover these attractions. Adolescents may also react with shame from their own internalized values and judge the attractions as deviant or unhealthy.

As adolescents attempt to understand themselves and how they fit into their society, various coping strategies are employed. Out of fear of discovery, some adolescents withdraw physically and emotionally from those around them. In a 1987 study, Hetrick and Martin discovered that the major reason for seeking mental health services was a sense of isolation from family and peers. They also found that 5% of those seeking counseling used drugs. Other teens strive for athletic or academic overachievement, perfectionism, or over-involvement in extracurricular activities. As a "reaction formation against unacceptable thoughts and attractions," some adolescent girls "may exaggerate their heterosexuality and engage in promiscuous behavior, even becoming pregnant . . ." (Fontaine and Hammond 1996). Many avoid issues involving sexual identity until adulthood and experience a delayed social and sexual adolescence. Some date opposite-sex partners to avoid gossip and in hopes of "curing" themselves of their desires. Others marry at a young age and quickly have children. Some others remain celibate. Some turn to religion with hopes of eradicating sexual thoughts (Johnson and Johnson 2000).

A sense of community with others is vital to psychological well-being. Other minorities in society are based on race or culture. Children in these groups have their parents or other family members to protect and nurture them. Most adolescents with a sexual identity that differs from heterosexuality do not have that luxury. Many never have met, or are unaware they have met, others like them. Sexual minority adults who could be positive role models avoid mentoring young people out of fear they will be accused of "recruiting members." Isolation can be quite corrosive to anyone's self-esteem and may lead individuals to accept the prevailing homophobia, or at least heterosexism, that surrounds them. Popular myths that all gay persons are promiscuous and incapable of forming loving relationships strongly conflict with many young peoples' desire to re-create for themselves families like the ones in which they live. Further, the prevailing culture focuses on the sexual component of sexual minorities' orientation and excludes feelings of attraction, love, and companionship. As a result, "gay adolescents tend to view themselves as the problem, and fear the ostracism to which revealing their 'difference' might lead" (Anderson 1987, p. 177).

The AIDS epidemic has also inhibited the development of gay men. Fear of contracting AIDS, or of being identified with a population that many view as ill, has prevented some men from healthy sexual development. These men deny themselves sexual relationships out of fear of AIDS:

> The AIDS epidemic and increasing homophobia are producing developmental lags in some young gay men by adding to the perception that their sexuality is sinful, sick, or simply a matter of lust. It has caused some men to be afraid to express themselves as gay, depriving these young adults of the kind of experimentation necessary to understand themselves as men capable of a full and responsive sexuality in close and mutually loving relationships. (Isay 1989, p. 68)

Impact of Victimization on Identity Development

A growing body of quantitative research explores the needs of sexual minority youth with a particular interest in documenting harassment and victimization. The researchers of the Safe Schools Coalition of Washington reviewed the findings of eight population-based studies from 1987 to 1997 that surveyed a total of 83,042 middle and high school students (of all sexual orientations) around the United States (Reis and Saewyc 1999). Five of the relevant studies are part of the national Youth Risk Behavior Survey (YRBS) coordinated by the Centers for Disease Control and Prevention (CDC).

Although the researchers caution in making generalizations from the data because of the limitations of the studies, including the absence of homeless and out-of-school youth in these surveys, the data give an evolving understanding of the experiences of high school students who already self-identify as gay, lesbian, or bisexual, who already have had same-gender sexual experiences, or who already feel attracted to people of their own gender. In particular, the challenges of coming out in an atmosphere that includes verbal and physical harassment, threats, and victimization may impact the youth's self-esteem, academic performance, risk-taking behavior, and overall mental health.

Reis and Saewyc (1999, p. 21) conclude:

> The findings of these quantitative studies, especially in combination with one another, are quite conclusive about a number of things:
>
> 1. There are sexual minority children and youth in every community and every school district, as well as children who experience anti-gay bullying. If a District has 5,000 students,
>   a. At least 2% (100 teens) and possibly as many as 4.5% (225 teens) will probably identify as gay, lesbian or bisexual when they are in high school,
>   b. And at least 4.9% (245 teens) and perhaps as many as 8.1% (405 teens) will probably say, by the time they are in high school, that they have been harassed because someone thought they were gay.
> 2. Sexual minority youth in general, as well as heterosexual youth who are harassed for being perceived to be gay,
>   a. Are at increase risk for also being threatened and assaulted,

b. Are disproportionately likely to have been harmed at home (sexually and/or physically abused),

c. Are disproportionately likely to be fearful for their safety at school, to the point of skipping whole days because of it, and

d. Are significantly more likely than their heterosexual, non-harassed peers to engage in self-endangering behaviors such as:

    i. Abusing alcohol and other drugs;

    ii. Becoming pregnant or getting someone pregnant;

    iii. Vomiting or taking laxatives to lose weight, and/or

    iv. Thinking about, planning and attempting suicide.

These data reflect the challenges for sexual minority youths in developing a healthy identity in an atmosphere that might appear to be relatively supportive on its surface. However, schools have only recently begun to address bullying, harassment, and school violence. Even fewer schools incorporate education and support that specifically addresses sexual minority youth.

Self-Disclosure of Sexual Orientation

Despite the many hurdles and fears a young person may have over self-disclosure, many adolescents begin the process of telling others about their desires. There is some indication that some youth are announcing their sexual identities at an earlier age than was the case even 10 years ago.

Responses to Self-Disclosure

The responses these youth receive to their self-disclosure vary a great deal from person to person. According to recent data, one of every three gay youth experiences verbal abuse from family members, one of four receives physical abuse from peers at school, and one of three has attempted suicide (D'Augelli 1998). The Hetrick-Martin Institute estimates that 25% of gay youth are thrown out of their homes by their parents after coming out (Godfried and Godfried 2001). In the Los Angeles area, approximately

18% of homeless youth are gay, lesbian, or bisexual (Unger et al. 1997). Approximately 40% lose at least one friend after disclosure (D'Augelli and Hershberger 1993; Remafredi 1987).

Similar problems continue into college. In a study of 121 sex-ual minority students conducted at a large university in 1992 (D'Augelli 1992), 75% received verbal insults; 27% were threat-ened with physical violence, 22% were chased or followed, and 5% had suffered some form of physical abuse; and 22% reported harassment from their roommates. Perhaps it is not surprising that the same study found that 70% of sexual minorities hid their orientation from their roommates and 80% hid their orientation from other students.

A 1993 study at Yale University found that 42% of sexual minority students had been physically abused. Almost 20% had been assaulted two or more times, presumably because of their sexual orientation (Herek 1993).

Parental Acceptance

Many of the stressors that sexual minority adolescents face can be mitigated by an adequate support network. In particular, parents can be a great resource for children if they are supportive and understanding, or at least tolerant, of what their child is experi-encing. A 1995 study found that family support significantly re-duced the stress and symptoms of victimization experienced by gay teenagers (Hershberger and D'Augelli 1995). Parish and McCluskey (1992) found a correlation between the love and ac-ceptance provided by parents and the improved self-image and self-esteem of their children. A 1989 study of lesbian teenagers found that the youth were more comfortable with their sexuality when both parents were accepting and that the mother's accep-tance was particularly important; a similar study of gay men found that healthy self-esteem was associated with support from both parents (Savin-Williams 1989).

That parental acceptance is an important part of healthy de-velopment should come as no surprise. As Fontaine and Ham-mond (1996) noted, "[L]esbian and gay adolescents have the same needs for economic, physical, and emotional dependence and nurturance from parents as do heterosexual adolescents." However, fear of parental rejection prevents many teens from revealing their sexual orientation to their parents. One study found that gay male adolescents were less likely to come out to their parents if they grew up in a family with more traditional values. Those values were defined as the importance of religion, emphasis on marriage and having children, and use of a non-English language at home (Newman and Muzzonigro 1993).

For those who do risk telling their parents, the results are somewhat encouraging. Although some parents react by ostracizing their children or becoming abusive, many react in a much more positive way. In a study of adult gay men by Cramer and Roach (1988), 70% expected their relationship with their parents to worsen after coming out to them. In contrast, among gay men who did tell their fathers they were gay, only 42% experienced a deterioration in their relationship. Similarly, the less mothers and fathers were perceived to know, the more negative were the anticipated responses (D'Augelli and Hershberger 1993). Cramer and Roach (1988) found that revelation did initially cause stress in parent-child relationships but that over time the relationships tended to recover and sometimes became stronger than ever.

Often parents feel conflicted between the love they have for their child and their own internalized prejudice and fear of homosexual persons or other sexual minorities. If unprepared for their child's revelation, parents will likely react with some initial shock. That shock is followed by a process of gradually working through the conflict, with various degrees of resolution over time. A 1987 study of 111 families found that 48% had a "Loving, Denial" relationship, characterized by a positive relationship between parent and child, but the parents were unable to discuss their child's sexual orientation with others; 36% experienced a "Resentful, Denial" relationship, in which little contact occurred between parents and their child; 5% received "Hostile Recognition" and nonacceptance, leading to total estrangement; and 11% experienced "Loving Open" relationships with their parents, with the parents being accepting and also positive in sharing information about their child's sexual orientation with others (Muller 1987).

In general, it is likely that parents will have difficulty adjusting to their child's sexual orientation once it is revealed to them. Even supportive parents may feel confused about how to manage their child's development effectively, because the traditional rules of child-rearing may no longer apply. For example, to which same-sex friends might their child be attracted? Are sleepovers okay? What dating rules should apply?

Other Support

Other supports are also important for healthy development. The literature strongly encourages sexual minority youth to find positive images of themselves in the media and in other resources. The Internet can be an avenue to find others and discuss problems and offer support online. Sexual minority youth organizations can, if possible, offer counseling, support, and the opportunity to socialize with other sexual minority peers. Counselors and therapists can direct these youth to resources that offer a more realistic understanding of themselves. The formation of Gay Straight Alliances has occurred at some schools.

Sexual Activity and Dating

Issues of sexual activity and dating among sexual minority youth is in some ways more difficult to discuss. Only a handful of studies on these issues occurred in the 1970s, 1980s, and early 1990s. The earlier studies involved surveying gay and lesbian adults about recollections of their adolescence. In 1988 and 1989, lesbian, gay male, and bisexual youth were surveyed in Chicago on initial awareness of same-sex attraction, fantasy, and first sexual activity with either same or opposite sex partners (Boxer 1988; Boxer et al. 1989). Using different methodology from that used in earlier research, this study found that awareness of same-sex attraction, activity, and disclosure happened earlier than was found in earlier research. A survey of gay male college students in 1991 showed similar results. On average, the respondents became aware of same-sex feelings by age 11, had their first same-sex sexual experience 4.5 years later, identified themselves as gay just prior to entering college, and disclosed their orientation to someone else by age 19 (D'Augelli 1991). Further, D'Augelli (1991), examining whether self-identification as gay correlated with same-sex sexual activity, found that 11% of respondents had same-sex encounters before self-labeling, 8% simultaneously with self-labeling, and 75% after self-labeling.

Only a few studies have specifically examined the dating habits of sexual minority youth. The research that has been done suggests that these youth engage in heterosexual dating and heterosexual sexual activity (Bell and Weinberg 1981; Boxer et al. 1989; Gundlach and Riess 1968; Saghir and Robins 1973; Savin-Williams 1990; Schafer 1976; Sears 1991; Spada 1979; Troiden and Goode 1980; Weinberg and Williams 1974). Again, the earlier studies were conducted with adults by means of retrospective analysis, and the later studies (those by Boxer et al., Savin-Williams, and Sears) involved direct polling of adolescents. The reasons frequently cited for heterosexual dating and sexual activity were denial of same-sex feelings, curiosity, a desire to conform to societal norms, and an attempt to reduce personal stress around coming-out issues (Savin-Williams 1990). When asked how they experienced their opposite-sex sexual experiences, youth responded that it was "sex without feelings"—that it felt unnatural and lacked emotional intensity.

In a 1991 study of sexual minority youth in the southern United States, 90% had dated opposite-sex partners, and 25% had also dated someone of the same sex. However, the same-sex dates were characterized as brief encounters with little emotional commitment and occurred in secrecy (Sears 1991). D'Augelli (1991) surveyed 61 college males and found that half were in "partnered" relationships, which on average began at age 19. Almost half of those relationships lasted for longer than 6 months. Savin-Williams (1990), in similar research, found that just over 65% of males and 80% of females reported a same-sex romantic relationship in high school or college. Savin-Williams also found that lesbian and bisexual women began romantic relationships at an earlier age, had more relationships, and had longer-lasting relationships than their male peers.

Savin-Williams (1990) found that gay and bisexual male

youth who had romantic relationships with boys were more likely to have had a number of love affairs, more likely to be in a current relationship, and had high self-esteem. They were not, however, more likely to be publicly "out." Similarly, a study of lesbian youth found a high correlation between involvement in a lesbian relationship and high self-esteem, self-acceptance, and social support (Rothblum 1990). In contrast, Coleman (1989) found that gay male youth who were denied opportunities for peer dating and socialization turned to anonymous sexual encounters with adults; these youths were purported to be at increased risk for sexually transmitted diseases, including HIV infection.

Sexual Minority Youth in Other Minority Groups

Even less is known about the unique experiences of sexual minority youth who also belong to other minority groups based on race, religion, or another reason. In most ethnic minority cultures, deviance from the heterosexual norm is even less tolerated than it is by society in general. These youth must manage more than one stigmatized identity, which increases their risk for stress and vulnerability to rejection. They have to deal with stereotypes about gender and sex roles, child-rearing, and religious values particular to the culture in which they are raised. They may also struggle with varying degrees of assimilation into mainstream culture (Ryan and Futterman 1997). Further, when they turn to the lesbian and gay subculture for support, they are sometimes met with the same ethnic or cultural prejudices held by the dominant society. The only available statistical finding on the impact of ethnic diversity is that African American and Native American lesbians have more children than do white lesbians (Greene 1994).

Bisexual and Transgender Youth

Research suggests that bisexual youth face different developmental issues than their gay and lesbian counterparts. Also, the term *bisexual* is sometimes self-applied by individuals who later identify as gay male or lesbian. In such cases, the self-labeling is seen as a part of the "coming out" process and is not regarded as a true bisexual identity. Though they may experiment with same- and opposite-sex partners during adolescence, most bisexual youth tend to identify as heterosexual until their mid to late 20s. Some feel misunderstood by and estranged from the gay and lesbian communities. These individuals may feel pressure from the heterosexual and homosexual worlds to conform to one group or the other (Fox 1991; Klein 1993; Rust 1993; Weinberg et al. 1994).

The majority of transgender persons are heterosexual in their sexual orientation but may identify as homosexual, heterosexual, bisexual, or asexual. However, they often turn to the gay and lesbian communities for support (Feinberg 1996). Transgender youth often face more overt hostility than their gay and lesbian counterparts because of their gender-atypical behavior. Males in particular are at high risk for verbal and physical abuse. The exact number of transgender people is unknown. It is estimated that 1 in 30,000 males and 1 in 100,000 females seek help at gender identity clinics. Most who seek help do not want sex reassignment surgery. Among those who seek help, high rates of substance abuse, attempted suicide, and psychiatric problems are reported. Little is known about transgender persons who do not use gender identity clinics. Little research has occurred with transgender youth and their developmental issues.

References

Anderson D: Family and peer relations of gay adolescents. Adolesc Psychiatry 14:162–178, 1987

Beaty L: Identity development of homosexual youth and parental and familial influences on the coming out process. Adolescence 34:597–601, 1999

Bell A, Weinberg M, Hammersmith S: Sexual Preference: Its Development in Men and Women. Bloomington, Indiana University Press, 1981

Boxer A: Betwixt and between: developmental discontinuities of gay and lesbian youth. Paper presented at the biennial meeting of the Society for Research on Adolescence, Alexandria, Va, April 1988

Boxer A, Cook J, Herdt G: First homosexual and heterosexual experiences reported by gay and lesbian youth in an urban community. Paper presented at the annual meeting of the American Sociological Association, San Francisco, CA, August 1989

Cass V: Homosexual identity formation: a theoretical model. J Homosex 4:219–235, 1979

Cass V: Sexual orientation identity formation: a Western phenomenon, in Textbook of Homosexuality and Mental Health. Edited by Cabaj R, Stein T. Washington, DC, American Psychiatric Press, 1996, pp 227–251

Coleman E: Developmental stages of the coming out process, in Homosexuality and Psychotherapy. Edited by Gonsiorek JC. New York, Haworth, 1982, pp 31–44

Coleman E: The development of male prostitution activity among gay and bisexual adolescence. J Homosex 17:131–149, 1989

Cramer D, Roach A: Coming out to mom and dad: a study of gay males and their relationships with their parents. J Homosex 15:79–91, 1988

D'Augelli A: Gay men in college: identity processes and adaptations. Journal of College Student Development 32:140–146, 1991

D'Augelli A: Lesbian and gay male undergraduates' experiences of harassment and fear on campus. Journal of Interpersonal Violence 7:383–395, 1992

D'Augelli A: Developmental implications of victimization of lesbian, gay, and bisexual youths, in Stigma and Sexual Orientation: Understanding Prejudice Against Lesbians, Gay Men, and Bisexuals. Edited by Herek GM. Thousand Oaks, CA, Sage, 1998, pp 187–210

D'Augelli A, Hershberger S: Lesbian, gay, and bisexual youth in community settings: personal challenges and mental health problems. Am J Community Psychol 21:421–448, 1993

Feinberg L: Transgender Warriors. Boston, MA, Beacon Press, 1996

Fontaine J, Hammond N: Counseling issues with gay and lesbian adolescents. Adolescence 31:817–830, 1996

Fox R: Coming out bisexual: identity, behavior and sexual orientation self-disclosure. Unpublished doctoral dissertation, California Institute of Integral Studies, 1991

Godfried M, Godfried A: The importance of parental support in the lives of gay, lesbian, and bisexual individuals. JCLP/In Session: Psychotherapy in Practice 57:681–693, 2001

Greene B: Lesbian women of color: triple jeopardy, in Women of Color: Integrating Ethnic and Gender Identities in Psychotherapy. Edited by Comas-Diaz L, Greene B. New York, Guilford, 1994, pp 389–427

Gundlach R, Riess B: Self and sexual identity in the female: a study of female homosexuals, in New Directions in Mental Health. Edited by Riess BF. New York, Grune & Stratton, 1968, pp 205–231

Herek G: Documenting prejudice against lesbians and gay men on campus: the Yale Sexual Orientation Study. J Homosex 25:15–30, 1993

Hershberger S, D'Augelli A: The consequences of victimization on the mental health and suicidality of lesbian, gay, and bisexual youth. Dev Psychol 31:65–74, 1995

Hetrick E, Martin A: Developmental issues and their resolution for gay and lesbian adolescents. J Homosex 14:25–43, 1987

Isay R: Fathers and their homosexually inclined sons in childhood. Psychoanal Study Child 42:275–284, 1987

Isay R: Being Homosexual: Gay Men and Their Development. Northvale, NJ, Jason Aronson, 1989

Isay R: The development of sexual identity in homosexual men, in The Course of Life, Vol 4: Adolescence. Edited by Greenspan SI, Pollock GH. Madison, CT, International Universities Press, 1991, pp 469–492

Johnson C, Johnson K: High-risk behavior among gay adolescents: implications for treatment and support. Adolescence 35:619–637, 2000

Klein F: The Bisexual Option, 2nd Edition. New York, Harrington Park Press, 1993

Muller A: Parents Matter: Parents' Relationships With Lesbian Daughters and Gay Sons. Tallahassee, FL, Naiad Press, 1987

Newman, B, Muzzonigro P: The effects of traditional family values on the coming out process of gay male adolescents. Adolescence 28:213–226, 1993

Parish T, McCluskey J: The relationship between parenting styles and young adults' self-concepts and evaluations of parents. Adolescence 27:915–918, 1992

Reis B, Saewyc E: Eighty-three thousand youth: selected findings of eight population based studies. Safe Schools Coalition of Washington, May 1999. Available at: http://www.safeschoolscoalition.org/83000youth.pdf. (pp. 1–29)

Remafredi G: Adolescent homosexuality: psychosocial and medical implications. Pediatrics 79:331–337, 1987

Rothblum E: Depression among lesbians: an invisible and unresearched phenomenon. Journal of Gay and Lesbian Psychotherapy 1:67–87, 1990

Rotherham-Borus MJ, Fernandez MI: Sexual orientation and developmental challenges experienced by gay and lesbian youths. Suicide Life Threat Behav 25(suppl):26–34, 1995

Rust P: "Coming out" in the age of social constructionism: sexual identity formation among lesbian and bisexual women. Gender and Society 7(1):50–77, 1993

Ryan C, Futterman D: Lesbian and gay youth: care and counseling. Adolesc Med 8(2):207–374, 1997

Saghir M, Robins E: Male and Female Homosexuality. Baltimore, MD, Williams & Wilkins, 1973

Savin-Williams R: Coming out to parents and self-esteem among gay and lesbian youths. J Homosex 18:1–35, 1989

Savin-Williams R: Gay and Lesbian Youth: Expressions of Identity. Washington, DC, Hemisphere, 1990

Schafer S: Sexual and social problems of lesbians. Journal of Sex Research 12:50–69, 1976

Sears J: Growing Up Gay in the South: Race, Gender and Journeys of the Spirit. New York, Harrington Park Press, 1991

Siegel S, Lowe E: Unchartered Lives: Understanding the Life Passages of Gay Men. New York, Dutton, 1994

Spada J: The Spada Report: The Newest Survey of Gay Male Sexuality. New York, New American Library, 1979

Telljohann S, Price J: A qualitative examination of adolescent homosexuals' life experiences: ramifications for secondary school personnel. J Homosex 26:41–56, 1993

Troiden RR: Becoming homosexual: a model of gay identity acquisition. Psychiatry 42:362–373, 1979

Troiden R, Goode E: Variables related to the acquisition of a gay identity. J Homosex 5:383–392, 1980

Unger J, Kipke M, Simon T, et al: Homeless youths and young adults in Los Angeles: prevalence of mental health problems and the relationship between mental health and substance abuse disorders. American Journal of Community Psychology 25:371–394, 1997

Weinberg M, Williams C: Male Homosexuals: Their Problems and Adaptations. New York, Penguin Books, 1974

Weinberg M, Williams C, Pryor D: Dual Attraction: Understanding Bisexuality. New York, Oxford University Press, 1994

Zera D: Coming of age in a heterosexist world: the development of gay and lesbian adolescents. Adolescence 27:849–854, 1992

Chapter 2

Aging and
Sexual Orientation

Douglas C. Kimmel, Ph.D.

If one thinks of the extended family—in-laws, cousins, nieces, nephews, aunts, uncles, brothers, sisters, children, and the grand-parents' relatives—most families include diversity in terms of ethnic or racial background and sexual orientation. This fact is useful to keep in mind when beginning a discussion of issues related to diversity. Most mental health practitioners and profes-sionals who work with the elderly have a relative or friend who is known or thought to be lesbian, gay, or bisexual. Thus, when we address sexual orientation issues, we are not talking about some peculiar group of strangers, but persons who are our friends and family members.

Moreover, when one thinks of sexual orientation, it is impor-tant to note that much more is involved than sex. Consider the following script that may be used to begin a training session on sexual orientation issues for staff in an extended care facility and those providing in-home services.

> Think of the activity you most enjoy doing, whether it is paint-ing, playing golf, hunting, cooking, traveling, or playing with your grandchildren. . . .
>
> Now think of the person or people you love the most and how important they are to you. . . .
>
> Now imagine that you fell and broke a hip and wound up in a hospital and then in a nursing home for rehabilitation—hopefully for only a few weeks until you can return home.
>
> However, in that nursing home you cannot let *anyone* know your favorite activity, or the person or people you love the most. You cannot mention anything about them.

This is the situation for most lesbian, gay, and bisexual persons, because often others can infer one's sexual orientation from important activities and loved persons. Sexual orientation involves the books we read, our community activities, and our friendships.

Finally, imagine that you are going home with a home health aide whom you do not know. As you think about the way you left your home, you recall all the photos of your loved persons on the shelf and all the signs of your favorite activity scattered around the house. How are you going to explain them to your new aide?

To understand the situation of older lesbian, gay, and bisexual persons, we need to consider the effects of having a *concealed social stigma* that may or may not be revealed or discovered. Often when such stigma is discovered, it operates as a kind of *master status* that overwhelms all other dimension of social status and roles. In a sense, old age also operates as a master status.

Historical Background of the Current Cohorts of Older Adults

Lesbians, bisexual persons, and gay men over age 85 in 2002—the fastest growing cohort in the United States today—were born before 1917; they would have reached their twenty-first birthday by 1938 and probably served in the armed forces during World War II, where many of them discovered the significance of their sexual orientation (Berube 1990). Often it included a positive discovery of others who shared their same-sex attraction and was, in many ways, the beginning of the modern gay, bisexual, and lesbian community. For others, however, it was a devastating experience, sometimes resulting in a "blue paper" discharge that hindered their return to American society and the workforce; it even prevented their access to GI benefits in many cases (Loughery 1998).

The cohorts over age 70 in 2002 were born before 1932 and would have been over age 21 when President Eisenhower issued executive order #10450 in 1953 that encouraged dismissing homosexuals from government jobs. This order coincided with the anti-Communist crusade by Senator McCarthy and others. However, as Loughery (1998) notes, "the number of men and women dismissed for sexual reasons far exceeds—by any estimates—the number dismissed for real or alleged involvement with the Communist Party" (p. 208). The discovery and exposure of gay men was not limited to government employees. In 1955 a witchhunt began in Boise, Idaho, that led to almost 1,500 men being interviewed by police about their sexuality, and 10 were sent to prison, some for having homosexual sex with consenting adults (Gerassi 1966; Loughery 1998). In 1958–1959, a 6-month investigation of homosexuals took place at the University of Florida.

> Married or single, members of the English, speech, music, education, and science departments, they were as different as any such group would be, ranging in age from their thirties to their late fifties. Several had published significantly in their fields, and almost all were tenured. Two, including an assistant dean, were recent Fulbright scholars, and to judge from the recently opened records in the Florida State Archives, every one of the sixteen who was later fired had been evaluated as a capable, even outstanding teacher. (Loughery 1998, p. 247)

Meanwhile, the Mattachine Society, a pioneer organization providing support and education about homosexuality, held a national conference in Denver, Colorado, in 1959 that was reported in the *Denver Post* on September 4–6. The local organizer was later arrested, had his home searched, was jailed for 60 days, and lost his job. It was not until a U.S. Supreme Court decision in January 1958 that lesbian and gay publications such as the *Mattachine Review* could be delivered by the post office and were not considered obscene (Loughery 1998).

The current generation of persons over age 65 experienced this repressive period during their adult years. It should not be surprising to find that this cohort of older persons value discretion and often do not disclose their sexual orientation unless they feel it is necessary and safe to do so. This generation also grew up during the emergence of psychiatric views of homosexuality that viewed it as a pathological condition instead of sinful or criminal behavior. Although Freud (1935/1951) wrote an American mother that "[h]omosexuality . . . cannot be classified as an illness; we consider it to be a variation of the sexual function . . .," his idea that everyone was inherently bisexual led to unexpected results: As Loughery (1998) noted, "Disastrously, the acceptance of Freud's assertion that homosexual desire was an innate capacity shared by all men and women led not to the encouragement of tolerance or benign neglect, but to the alarmist notion that greater vigilance was the answer. Beware the dominant mother, take heed of the passive father: perversion begins at home" (p. 114).

For the current generation of middle-aged adults (ages 50–65), two distinct groups may be noted. The first group is made up of those whose lives were influenced by the modern gay, lesbian, bisexual, and transgender movement that became visible after the police raid on the Stonewall Inn bar in New York City in June 1969 began to be celebrated annually—primarily those born during the postwar "baby boom." The other group consists of those who were born prior to the end of the war, who would have been over age 24 at the time of the Stonewall events or who were relatively unaware of this cultural paradigm shift because of isolation or other reasons.

Each of these cohorts grew older during a period of rapid social change and, like a caravan of distinct groups, was differentially affected by the events of those years. The 1970s were clearly transitional years for the gay, lesbian, bisexual, and transgender movement, as their visibility increased, the women's movement called attention to gender issues, and significant progress was made toward removing the stigma of mental illness from homosexuality. The decade of the 1980s was marked by the HIV/AIDS epidemic, which had profound demographic as well as psychological effects on the cohort of survivors. The economic boom of the 1990s has probably affected retirement rates and, among other benefits, has led to the development of gay, lesbian, bisexual, and transgender retirement and assisted-living facilities in a few local areas.

It may be fair to conclude that the current population of older persons in the gay, lesbian, bisexual, and transgender communities is even more diverse than in the general population because of the uniqueness of their developmental experience as a sexual minority.

Aging Gay, Lesbian, Bisexual, and Transgender Persons as a Stigmatized Sexual Minority: Theoretical Models and Empirical Data

Sexual orientation cuts across the population in ways that are similar to the ways age cuts across the population: generalizations about gay men and lesbians are as risky as those about persons over age 65 or over age 85. In this chapter, both dimensions of diversity—age and sexual orientation—are considered. The result is very complex. Ethnic and racial differences, social class and educational background, health, income, and attention to well-being are as important variables in gay, lesbian, bisexual, and transgender aging as they are in aging in the general population. In addition, the cohort differences and personal experiential differences make generalization about older gay, lesbian, bisexual, and transgender persons extremely difficult. The use of the following three theoretical models can, however, shed some light on these issues: managing a concealable stigma, minority stress and resilience, and coping with multiple minority statuses. Each is discussed in turn.

Survival of the Fittest: Crisis Competence or Walking Wounded

Living with a concealed stigma, such as a minority sexual orientation, can be a heavy burden, especially if one's family or friends are not aware of the secret. Such situations are not rare in our society: persons who are hearing impaired, diabetic, or of mixed parentage may have similar experiences. Murphy-Shigematsu (1999) studied children in Japan of mixed Asian ancestry and concluded: "Some endure considerable and constant psychological stress in maintaining their secret. They live with the awareness that they are not presenting themselves honestly to others. . . . In a society like Japan's, where the presentation of self is extremely controlled and self-censored, and where being different is a major cause of exclusion, there is good reason for the great fear of going public" (p. 492). Similar tensions exist for many older lesbians, gay men, and bisexual persons, who often live a kind of double life, or have developed an identity wherein they are "gay" only in a small portion of their lives—perhaps only when they are actively participating in homosexual activity of some type. Many do not disclose their secret to family, friends, or co-workers.

Research studies of older gay men and lesbians can focus only on *survivors* who have lived long enough to be included in the sample age group. Since longitudinal data do not exist, we do not know what proportion of young gay men, lesbians, bisexual persons, and transgender persons actually grow old. Nor do we know the conditions that led to their death. All we can conclude is that the present generation of older persons in the community did not die earlier from infectious diseases, accidents, alcoholism, cancer, cardiovascular disease, HIV/AIDS, substance abuse, suicide, or anything else; nor are they in prison or long-term care institutions. These facts are often overlooked in cross-sectional studies of elderly persons and tend to skew the data toward the more robust and mainstream populations. Therefore, each generation of older persons is unique, and results cannot be generalized directly to future generations of older persons, who may benefit from better health care, lower morbidity in earlier life, and different social and environmental conditions.

Most studies of older lesbians and gay men have focused on persons who are involved in the gay, lesbian, bisexual, and transgender communities in some way and thus are not representative of older persons who are erotically attracted to others of the same sex. These studies have found that those persons are aging in relatively good physical and mental health; they do not fit the stereotype of lonely, depressed, and isolated old "queens" and "dykes" portrayed in the popular idea that gay and lesbian life is only for the young (Berger and Kelly 1996; Dorfman et al. 1995; Friend 1990; Quam and Whitford 1992).

Representative samples are occasionally available and provide a useful demographic portrait. One study in Australia of gay men found that more than half of those over age 50 lived alone—a greater proportion than in the younger age groups; older gay men were overrepresented in rural areas and less likely to live in predominantly gay areas, and they were more likely than younger gay men to have been married and to have children (Van de Ven et al. 1997).

Several studies have reported the development of a kind of *crisis competence* among many of the respondents (Kimmel 1978, 1995). In an early report, Weinberg and Williams (1974) noted that the older male homosexuals in their study were, in some respects, better adjusted then the younger homosexual men. They suggested that "[h]omosexuals . . . may face their major 'discontinuity' crisis at an earlier age, for example, identity crises during early adulthood. . . . By middle age, however, the homosexual may have grown accustomed to such experiences and, as a result, not find them so disturbing" (p. 220, footnote). Disclosing one's sexual orientation, confronting the reactions of family members or friends, managing the stigma of being unmarried or surviving a divorce, sharing a home or apartment with a lover of the same sex, and dealing with verbal or even physical abuse can develop one's coping skills for managing the concealable stigma and the resulting master status if it is exposed.

These same conditions can lead to overwhelming stress, however, so that instead of leading to crisis competence, they may lead to maladaptive responses and psychological deterioration (Lee 1991). It is likely that the positive or negative outcome is the result of the type of stressful event, preexisting coping skills, economic resources, and personal resilience. Peer support, positive role models, family support, absence of history of previous trauma or abuse, effective coping skills, and a well-developed sense of personal identity would be expected to promote the development of crisis competence.

Looking at data for older lesbians and gay men, we see signs of both crisis competence and the long-term effects of the social stigma of homosexuality. One of the largest studies to date (Grossman et al. 2001) used gay, lesbian, bisexual, and transgender organizations to recruit a nationwide sample of 416 lesbians, gay men, and bisexual persons over the age of 60; 71% were male and 29% were female, and 8% identified as bisexual. The vast majority (84%) said their mental health was good or excellent; 14% said it was fair, and only 2% reported it to be poor. Their self-rating of mental health was directly related to income and inversely related to reported victimization for their sexual orientation. Living with a domestic partner was associated with positive mental health and with a higher reported level of self-esteem. Self-esteem was also positively related to income and with a greater number of persons in their support networks; it was inversely related to experiences of victimization. Only 8% reported being depressed about being gay, lesbian, or bisexual; 9% said they had been to mental health counseling to stop their same-sex feelings; and 17% said they would prefer being heterosexual. Men reported more suicide thoughts related to their sexual orientation than did women. Overall, 10% said they considered suicide sometimes or often; 13% reported a suicide attempt, generally between the ages of 22 and 59. There was no relationship between age and reports of feeling lonely, although 27% said they lacked companionship and 13% said they felt isolated. Loneliness was inversely related to income and the number of people in their support group; it was directly related to having experienced victimization for their sexual orientation.

These findings indicate that older lesbians, gay men, and bisexual persons who are recruited from gay, lesbian, bisexual, and transgender organizations and friendship networks are coping relatively well, have some history of unusual stress related to their sexual orientation, and probably have developed some degree of crisis competence along the way. They do not seem to be, in general, a group of walking wounded individuals—although there surely are some who are, as Meris (2001) found in his interview study of homeless older gay men.

Minority Stress: Resilience or Pathological Adaptation

Psychological models of lesbian, gay, and bisexual issues have shifted from a focus on adaptation to a minority sexuality toward an emphasis on the effects of being a minority within a heterosexist society (Greene 2000). This approach emphasizes the similarities between sexual minorities and other marginalized groups and the absence of pathological effects as a result of the psychosocial stress involved in being a disadvantaged minority.

Despite overwhelming social adversity and ill treatment that make them psychologically more vulnerable than heterosexual men and women, lesbians and gay men as a group are not the harbingers of psychopathology that American mental health has historically depicted them to be. Given that they must routinely negotiate a hostile social climate, we might expect to see greater ranges of pathology among lesbians and gay men than their heterosexual counterparts. One might expect similar findings in other groups of disadvantaged people, where they are similarly absent. I suggest that this is no accident. Rather, it is a reflection of a special kind of resilience that may be found among many members of marginalized groups. (Greene 2000, p. 5)

Meyer (1995) identified three minority stressors that independently predict psychological distress for gay men and lesbians: internalized homophobia, perceived stigma, and actual prejudice events. Typical experiences of sexual minorities range from the petty and trivial hassles of daily life in a heterosexist society, where everyone is assumed to be heterosexual, to being the unknown butt of jokes about homosexuals or listening to the frequent use of the term "faggot" or "gay" attached to anything that is perceived to be negative or socially unacceptable. More serious is personal verbal harassment or physical attack. A telephone poll of a random sample in 15 major cities, which included a question about sexual orientation, found that among those who self-identified as gay, lesbian, or bisexual (n = 405), 74% had experienced verbal harassment and 32% had experienced physical harassment or damage to their property because of their sexual orientation; 85% of the lesbians, 76% of the gay men, and 60% of the bisexual persons reported they had experienced discrimination (Associated Press 2001). Similarly, in their study of persons over age 60, Grossman et al. (2001) found that over their lifetime 63% reported experiencing verbal abuse, 29% had been threatened with violence, 16% had been assaulted, 11% had had objects thrown at them, and 12% had been attacked with a weapon because of their sexual orientation; 29% had been threatened with disclosure of their sexual orientation. Men were more likely to report victimization than were women; those who were members of more gay, lesbian, bisexual, and transgender organizations or attended them regularly were more likely to report victimization. Higher income was associated with lower reported incidents of victimization.

Jones (1997) analyzed the resilience of African Americans in ways that Greene (2000) found parallel to the experience of lesbians, gay men, and bisexual persons. For example, distinctive communities of support (often involving secret subcultures), reliance on their own self-identity, and self-generated definition of their origins were important. Greene (2000) concluded:

> The process of independent self-construction allows healthy individuals to . . . correctly understand that their subordinate social position is not the simple result of cultural deficiency, poor or inadequate values, individual or group defect, or mother nature, as they have been told. Rather, social privilege can be recognized as a function of interlocking social systems of selective discrimination and selective patterned advantage that has been deliberately designed to maintain the balance of social power. (p. 9)

The two themes of *minority stress* and *resilience* have begun to receive more attention in psychological research. Taken together, they reframe the question of aging sexual minorities from one of isolated individuals needing care to one of a resilient group of individuals who have found effective ways of providing care to one another in the face of extraordinary stress as a minority group. The latter view focuses on what they have to offer each other and younger generations and on building on their strengths to meet future challenges. SAGE (Senior Action in a Gay Environment; http://www.sageusa.org) has been utilizing this resource since 1977 in providing a range of programs by and for older lesbian, gay, bisexual, and transgender persons in New York City.

This perspective of minority stress also provides a link between sexual minorities, ethnic and racial minorities, gender, class, and age discrimination. It raises the question as to whether these negative social positions increase minority stress in an additive way: whether *multiple minorities*, such as old, black, gay, and female, are four times as stressful as only one, or whether the effect might be exponential— 16 times more stressful, for example.

Multiple Minority Status: Additional Resources or Exponential Stressors

Audre Lorde (1990) wrote: "As a Black lesbian feminist comfortable with the many different ingredients of my identity, and a woman committed to racial and sexual freedom from oppression, I find I am constantly being encouraged to pluck some one aspect of myself and present this as the meaningful whole, eclipsing or denying other aspects of myself" (p. 285). With aging, the master status of "old age" takes over and eclipses all other aspects of the person. It is assumed that one is no longer sexual after "a certain age," that sexual orientation is no longer important, and that physical infirmities are the great equalizer of all social status differences. A visit to a nursing home will confirm that it is extremely difficult to retain the important aspects of one's previous identity and that being lesbian, gay, or bisexual is way down the list of relevant considerations.

Many ethnic lesbians and gay men report that adjusting to being a double minority is much more difficult than being either an ethnic minority or a sexual minority. It would be useful to have empirical research on the impact of multiple minority statuses. However, the simple experience of being an *outsider* in relation to some social system seems to be necessary, but not sufficient, to increase the coping skills needed to master the challenges conferred by a different minority status. A gay man, for example, is not necessarily able to understand the issues of ethnic minority gay men, and neither would necessarily be able to understand the issues of older gay men. Moreover, role models and learning successful coping strategies for minority identities do not seem to automatically provide resources for coping with additional minority identities. One hypothesis worth testing is as follows: Being a member of one or more stigmatized groups would give greater practical experience in coping with minority stress; thus, adding multiple minorities would add not only to the cumulative stress but also to the roster of coping skills. This line of research would aim to specify what variables lead to heightened levels of stress, the effectiveness of the coping skills, and resilience.

Families of Blood and Choice:
A Mosaic of Diversity and Options

Many lesbians, bisexual persons, and gay men are parents, grandparents, siblings, and important members of their extended families. Lesbians and gay men sometimes choose to become parents through adoption or alternative fertilization techniques. Some bisexual persons, lesbians, and gay men have been or are heterosexually married. Frequently, close relationships are maintained with the children and grandchildren even after divorce or separation. One study of older gay and bisexual men in Oslo, Norway, found that previously married men were better adjusted than those who were previously in a long-term same-sex relationship or had never had a relationship of longer than 2 years. In one case, a respondent's daughter had given him a cell phone so, if she had to work late, she could contact him so that he could pick up his granddaughter after school. Another man commented that this gay grandfather was lucky to have his daughter and her family because this man had only his cat for company. The men who seemed at greatest disadvantage were the ones who had had a long-term partner who had died (H. W. Kristiansen, "Older Gay Men in Norway: Past Lives and Present Concerns, unpublished paper, 2001).

Friendship networks often supplement the biological family as a source of support for gay men and lesbians. It is important that younger friends be included in the network, however, since friends from the same cohort are likely to become unavailable because of infirmities, geographic relocation for health reasons, or death. Many lesbians maintain close ties with some of the women they have loved in the past, and these networks can provide rich emotional support in later life. Gay and bisexual men tend to develop friendship networks around shared interests, which may include sexual activities, travel, or the arts; these networks can also last into old age. Heterosexual neighbors and friends are often included in these support networks. Women as well as men are frequently included in the close friendship networks of gay men and bisexual persons; in the past they may have provided a kind of "cover" for the men in a heterosexist world.

In Grossman et al.'s study of lesbians, gay men, and bisexual persons over age 60 described earlier (Grossman et al. 2000, 2001), friendship networks were found to be very important sources of social support. The respondents listed an average of 6.3 persons in their network: 90% listed close friends, 44% listed their life partners, 33% listed siblings, and 39% listed other relatives; social acquaintances were listed by 32%, co-workers by 15%, parents by 4%, and husbands or wives by 3%. About half of the people listed in the support networks were under age 60, and respondents were much older than the persons in their network—by an average of 10 years—for both women and men. Women listed more people in their networks and more women than did men; gay and bisexual men listed more gay and bisexual men than did women; bisexual respondents included more heterosexual persons in their networks than did gay and lesbian respondents. In general, persons who knew the respondents' sexual orientation provided more satisfying support, but participants were not any more satisfied with the support from others with the same sexual orientation. General social support was the most frequent type of support received (72%), followed by emotional support (62%), practical support (54%), advice and guidance (41%), and financial support (13%).

Support given by the respondent was not addressed in Grossman et al.'s study, but generally social support is a mutual process. Lesbians, gay men, and bisexual persons may also be providing help to aging parents or other relatives, and their biological families may look to them as valuable resources for emotional, financial, or specialized help. Social biological theory suggests that the presence of unmarried adults who could serve as surrogate parents probably gave such families a survival advantage; thus, homosexuality may have been an asset during human evolution (Wilson 1975). A similar argument has been made for the importance of having aged family members who remember how to survive historically rare events such as severe droughts (Mead 1970).

Long-term emotionally intimate relationships with a significant other person are important for many older persons. In the study reported above, Grossman et al. (2000) concluded: "Older adults who lived with a partner reported less loneliness and better physical and emotional health. This is partly because single LGB [lesbian, gay, bisexual] adults had significantly smaller support networks than partnered adults" (pp. P177–P178). Since there are no appropriate models for same-sex relationships, each couple develops their own pattern. For example, in an early study of 14 gay men between the ages of 55 and 81, 3 of the men were in relationships—of 30 years and 40 years for the first two men, respectively; the third had been with his current partner for 13 years following the death of his first, older, partner after a 25-year relationship. One couple lived together, and they were open to their neighbors and friends; in a second couple, the partners lived in separate apartments but spent a lot of time together; the third relationship had long periods of separation caused by business travel (Kimmel 1977). Similar diversity exists among lesbian couples (Peplau and Spalding 2000). The essential structure of same-sex relationships has been termed "peer friendships" and has been adopted as a model for some heterosexual dual-career couples (Schwartz 1994). The importance of children and grandchildren in the lives of older lesbians, bisexual persons, and gay men is a topic that deserves more attention in future research studies.

Ageism and Heterosexism: Similarities and Differences

It is interesting to note the similarities between the social construction of sexual orientation as a concealable sexual minority status that evokes discrimination and the social construction of aging in Western society. First, both social categories cut across all demographic groups, so that knowing that someone is "old" or "gay/lesbian/bisexual/transgender" gives no clue about any of his or her other social statuses. Second, both social categories are evaluated negatively and have such flagrant acts of discrimination associated with them that laws have been enacted to prevent such discrimination and words have been coined to describe the discrimination: *ageism* and *heterosexism*.

There are numerous similarities between aging and minority

sexual orientation, which may be summarized as follows. Both old age and minority sexual orientation

1. Have been the focus of an active search for biological origin, and possible cure, despite the fact that both are normal human characteristics.
2. Evoke irrational fear and avoidance in some people, who tend to avoid close contact and physical touching with both groups.
3. Evoke confusion with associated conditions: aging with senility or death; sexual orientation with gender identity or promiscuity.
4. Operate as a master status that obviates other relevant social positions and characteristics.
5. Are perceived as being best to avoid if possible; they are both dealt with by "Don't ask, don't tell" policies.
6. Are characterized more in terms of their perceived disadvantages than their advantages; losses are thought to exceed gains, strengths are seen only as compensations for weakness.
7. Are discriminatory views—ageism and heterosexism—that emphasize the importance of fertility and propagation as normative for everyone.
8. Are conferred a special status in some cultures, in which the individuals may be seen as having special powers resulting from their minority status.

In contrast, there are four clear differences between ageism and heterosexism:

1. Most people hope to become old one day; few hope to become a sexual minority.
2. No one blames the individual's choice, or his or her mother, for becoming old.
3. Families openly acknowledge and celebrate becoming older; few families celebrate their children coming out as lesbian, gay, bisexual, or transgender.
4. Churches and moral guardians do not urge older persons to avoid acting old, but they often urge sexual minorities to avoid acting on their erotic or romantic attractions.

Special Issues in Working With Aging Sexual Minorities

Treating older lesbians, gay men, bisexual persons, and transgender persons requires some understanding of the historical and social context of their lives. It also benefits from an awareness of the survivor skills they developed and used over the years to cope with their concealable social stigma. Are there areas of crisis competence or other coping skills that can be utilized to deal with their present concerns? Do previous failures to cope or being overwhelmed by victimization or discrimination affect their current situation?

It is often useful to reframe the issue from the individual to the social perspective and to focus on the minority stress that the person has endured. Are there lasting effects of this stress that can be dealt with in therapy? Consider the three aspects Meyer (1995) suggested: internalized homophobia, perceived stigma, and actual prejudice events. The final third of life may be an appropriate time to resolve these issues and put them to rest. Often after retirement, or in later life, the relevance of these issues is different or much reduced, compared with in earlier adulthood. Finally, strengthening resilience may help persons cope with the further social burden conferred by the additional minority status of old age.

Some therapists recommend group therapy as being especially helpful for older lesbians (Fassinger 1997) and gay men (Frost 1997). Attention needs also to be given to lesbians and gay men with chronic mental illness (Hellman 1996). The special issues of older transgender persons, including the long-term effects of hormone therapy, reactions of health care providers to persons with unusual or unexpected genitals, and the effects of the minority stress associated with having an unusual gender identity, are important (Donovan 2001).

The Council of Scientific Affairs of the American Medical Association (1996) noted: "Physicians in general have often expressed discomfort with gay men and lesbians. . . . In another study, published in 1991, 25% of the psychiatric faculty of a medical school admitted they were prejudiced against gay men and lesbians" (p. 1356). Some physicians and psychiatrists also experience discomfort or prejudice concerning older persons. Although it would be ideal to eliminate all such prejudice within oneself, it may be more practical to recognize the relevance of such prejudice and reduce its impact to the greatest extent possible. Referral to another professional who is more comfortable with the issues or to a service agency associated with the lesbian, gay, bisexual, and transgender communities may be the best treatment option.

At the most practical level, is your practice accessible and open to gay, lesbian, bisexual, and transgender persons? Do the forms patients are given respect minority sexual orientations and the nature of their significant relationships? Simply asking "marital status" can be offensive. Is your office a safe place for gay, lesbian, bisexual, and transgender persons and accessible for persons with physical disabilities? One of my colleagues moved her practice because her clients were being harassed for their gender nonconformity in the parking lot of her previous clinic location. Another needed a place with no stairs and doors that was accessible to persons with walkers and wheelchairs.

Are the hospitals and emergency clinics sensitive to gay, lesbian, bisexual, and transgender issues? Can they treat a "butch" lesbian, "effeminate" gay man, or intact transgender person with the same professional respect with which they would treat other local civic leaders? What is their policy with regard to "next of kin" visitation and medical decisions?

Which of your local skilled nursing facilities, boarding homes, or assisted living houses would you recommend for your patient's significant life partner? How would these facilities handle conjugal visits? Would they respect their preferences for visitation rights, medical directives, and bedside vigil at the end of life?

Issues about bereavement following the death of a long-term partner, adjustment to retirement, isolation, depression, and reactions to somatic problems are typical psychotherapy issues for older lesbian, gay, bisexual, and transgender persons. Kimmel (1977) discussed psychotherapy issues involving loneliness, desire for a younger sexual partner, problems in relationships, and concerns about aging for older gay men. Fassinger (1997) discussed frequent issues for older lesbians, including access to health care, isolation, relationship problems, bereavement, and issues about their children. In addition, multiple losses as a result of HIV infection, homelessness, and substance abuse have been reported among older gay men (Meris 2001).

In work with older lesbian, gay, bisexual, and transgender persons, it is useful to have a range of connections to the gay, lesbian, bisexual, and transgender communities and allies in various professions. A skilled lawyer is often needed to draft financial and health care documents that can survive a challenge by biological family members. An accountant may be helpful in arranging finances and property to ensure that the lack of legal marriage does not result in unnecessary tax penalties, loss of residence, or loss of income upon the death of a long-term partner. Social services and home health care may be necessary for some period of time during illness, especially if the person is living alone; those providing such services need to respect the person's life as a sexual minority and, ideally, include resources to maintain ties with the gay, lesbian, bisexual, and transgender communities.

Conclusion

Working with older persons can be unusually rewarding, because often they can teach us about the past in ways that are available only through oral history. In many cases, they are survivors who have developed coping skills that worked fairly well until some event late in life occurred with which they could not cope. In therapy, it is frequently much simpler to rebuild those coping skills, and thus restore the individual's ability to function competently, than it is to teach those same skills to a younger person who has never developed them. Finally, advances in health care are adding years to life and, in many cases, adding life to years. Psychiatry can play as important a role in this process as exercise, nutrition, or medications that restore sexual vigor.

References

American Medical Association, Council on Scientific Affairs: Health care needs of gay men and lesbians in the United States. JAMA 275: 1354–1359, 1996

Associated Press: Gays report a rise in public acceptance. November 13, 2001

Berger RM, Kelly JJ: Gay men and lesbians grown older, in Textbook of Homosexuality and Mental Health. Edited by Cabaj RP, Stein TS. Washington, DC, American Psychiatric Press, 1996, pp 305–316

Berube A: Coming Out Under Fire: The History of Gay Men and Women in World War Two. New York, Free Press, 1990

Donovan T: Being transgender and older: a first person account. Journal of Gay and Lesbian Social Services 13(4):19–22, 2001

Dorfman R, Walters K, Burke P, et al: Old, sad and alone: the myth of the aging homosexual. Journal of Gerontological Social Work 24(1–2):29–44, 1995

Fassinger RE: Issues in group work with older lesbians. Group 21:191–210, 1997

Freud S: Letter to an American mother (1935). Am J Psychiatry 107:786–787, 1951

Friend RA: Older lesbian and gay people: a theory of successful aging. J Homosex 20(3–4):99–118, 1990

Frost JC: Group psychotherapy with the aging gay male: treatment of choice. Group 21:267–285, 1997

Gerassi J: The Boys of Boise: Furor, Vice and Folly in an American City. New York, Macmillan, 1966

Greene B: Beyond heterosexism and across the cultural divide, in Education, Research, and Practice in Lesbian, Gay, Bisexual, and Transgendered Psychology: A Resource Manual. Edited by Greene B, Croom GL. Thousand Oaks, CA, Sage, 2000, pp 1–45

Grossman AH, D'Augelli AR, Hershberger SL: Social support networks of lesbian, gay, and bisexual adults 60 years of age and older. J Gerontol B Psychol Sci Soc Sci 55:P171–P179, 2000

Grossman AH, D'Augelli AR, O'Connell TS: Being lesbian, gay, bisexual, and 60 or older in North America. Journal of Gay and Lesbian Social Services 13(4):23–40, 2001

Hellman RE: Issues in the treatment of lesbian women and gay men with chronic mental illness. Psychiatr Serv 47:1093–1098, 1996

Jones F: Eloquent anonymity. Readings: A Journal of Reviews and Commentary in Mental Health 12(1):10–14, 1997

Kimmel DC: Psychotherapy and the older gay man. Psychotherapy 14: 386–393, 1977

Kimmel DC: Adult development and aging: a gay perspective. Journal of Social Issues 34(3):113–130, 1978

Kimmel DC: Lesbians and gay men also grow old, in Promoting Successful and Productive Aging. Edited by Bond LA, Cutler SJ, Grams A. Thousand Oaks, CA, Sage, 1995, pp 289–303

Lee JA: Foreword. J Homosex 20(3–4):xiii–xix, 1991

Lorde A: Age, race, class, and sex: women redefining difference, in Out There: Marginalization and Contemporary Cultures. Edited by Ferguson R, Gever M, Minh-ha, T, et al. New York, New Museum of Contemporary Art, 1990, pp 281–287

Loughery J: The Other Side of Silence: Men's Lives and Gay Identities: A Twentieth Century History. New York, Henry Holt, 1998

Mead M: Culture and Commitment: A Study of the Generation Gap. Garden City, NY, Doubleday, 1970

Meris D: Responding to the mental health and grief concerns of homeless HIV-infected gay men. Journal of Gay and Lesbian Social Services 13(4):103–111, 2001

Meyer I: Minority stress and mental health in gay men. J Health Soc Behav 7:9–25, 1995

Murphy-Shigematsu S: Clinical work with minorities in Japan: social and cultural context. Am J Orthopsychiatry 69:482–494, 1999

Peplau LA, Spalding LR: The close relationships of lesbians, gay men, and bisexuals, in Close Relationships: A Sourcebook. Edited by Hendrick C, Hendrick SS. Thousand Oaks, CA, Sage, 2000, pp 111–123

Quam JK, Whitford GS: Adaptation and age-related expectations of older gay and lesbian adults. Gerontologist 32:367–374, 1992

Schwartz P: Peer Marriage: How Love Between Equals Really Works. New York, Free Press, 1994

Van de Ven P, Rodden P, Crawford J, et al: A comparative demographic and sexual profile of older homosexually active men. J Sex Res 34: 349–360, 1997

Weinberg MS, Williams C: Male Homosexuals: Their Problems and Adaptations. New York, Oxford University Press, 1974

Wilson EO: Sociobiology: The New Synthesis. Cambridge, MA, Belknap Press/Harvard University Press, 1975

Chapter 3

Offering Psychiatric Opinion in Legal Proceedings When Lesbian or Gay Sexual Orientation Is an Issue

Richard G. Dudley Jr., M.D.

The visibility of self-identified lesbians and gay men has increased dramatically over the last two decades. In the United States, the response of individuals who are not gay or lesbian has been extremely varied, ranging from total acceptance, to tolerance, to absolute hatred. Similarly, there is a wide range of knowledge about and understanding of lesbians and gay men; so although some persons are quite familiar with these issues, others are ignorant of and/or have deeply held prejudices against lesbians and gay men.

Now, like other "minority groups" in the United States, lesbians and gay men are demanding equal rights and equal protections under the law. In addition, as is true with other groups, some lesbians and gay men have found themselves in trouble with the law. Consequently, there has been an increasing number of legal proceedings of all types involving lesbians and gay men, and in many of these legal matters the person's sexual orientation has been an issue. In a significant percentage of these cases, there has been a question before the court for which the opinion of a psychiatrist or other mental health professional has been sought; these professionals have testified in the role of forensic expert and/or as the lesbian or gay person's psychiatrist or therapist.

Although there are a growing number of legal proceedings in which a gay or lesbian sexual orientation is an issue, especially in major U.S. cities, the overall number is still so small that there has not yet been a major study or formal analysis of the forensic mental health issues involved in such cases. However, a review of some of these cases and discussions with attorneys and other mental health professionals who have been involved indicate that it is time to expand the dialogue on the issue of psychiatric opinion in legal proceedings when lesbian or gay sexual orientation is an issue.

There are at least two reasons why the dialogue should be expanded. The first reason is that the performance of a competent forensic mental health evaluation in such cases requires an in-depth understanding of lesbian and gay mental health issues. Therefore, mental health professionals must become more competent with regard to these issues before they perform such forensic evaluations. The second reason is that, given the limited knowledge of gay and lesbian mental health issues that many legal decision-makers have, mental health professionals who testify in cases involving gay men and lesbians must also be encouraged and trained to help legal decision-makers gain a richer understanding of gay and lesbian mental health issues. These two reasons underpin the need to expand the dialogue on offering psychiatric opinion in legal proceedings in which gay or lesbian sexual orientation is an issue and form the underlying motivations for writing this chapter.

Professional opinion is sought in legal proceedings when it is believed that a professional in a given field can help the decision-maker (be it a judge or a jury) comprehend an important aspect of the case that the decision-maker would otherwise be unable or less able to understand. For example, mental health professionals are regularly brought into legal proceedings to help decision-makers understand whether a defendant in a criminal proceeding was suffering from some type of psychiatric disorder that influenced the defendant's behavior in a certain way, or whether a plaintiff in a civil proceeding has been psychologically harmed as a result of something that the defendant did to the plaintiff. Of course, the value of professional opinion in legal proceedings depends, at least in part, on whether the professional does, in fact, have some special expertise to offer. Therefore, it is essential that psychiatrists and other mental health professionals become fully aware of underlying gay and lesbian mental health issues that inform our responses to the questions that may arise in these legal proceedings.

Even when psychiatrists and other mental health professionals have special expertise to offer, it is still quite likely that legal decision-makers may already have their own deeply held "theories" or beliefs about human behavior that can and often do significantly influence the outcome of legal proceedings. For example, legal decision-makers rarely believe that they can figure out the flight characteristics and effects of a bullet and then determine which alternative set of facts presented to them is most consistent with those findings. Therefore, they readily perceive the need for the help of a ballistics expert, and they tend to accept the opinion that the ballistics expert provides. On the other hand, a significant percentage of legal decision-makers believe they already know what is and is not good for children, or whether a specific individual accused of a crime is mentally ill or simply a bad person. Therefore, the opinions of a psychiatrist or other mental health professional are often viewed in the context of what decision-makers believe they already know. This can be the case regardless of whether a given decision-maker's understanding is in fact consistent with a theory of human behavior that is generally accepted within the mental health professions, or whether it can be more accurately described as an idiosyncratic notion or even an ill-informed bias.

In the most basic sense, a forensic mental health evaluation begins with the gathering of information, or "facts," that will form the basis for the evaluation. This usually involves an examination of the person(s) who is the focus of the legal proceeding, as well as interviews with additional relevant individuals and reviews of relevant records and documents. Then, by employing theories and/or empirical data that are accepted by the mental health professionals and relevant to the "facts," the mental health professional interprets the "facts" and renders a diagnosis and/or offers a dynamic formulation of the case. Since in most cases a diagnosis or dynamic formulation does not actually fully answer the legal questions asked, the mental health professional then employs more theories and/or empirical data to form an opinion about the legal questions.

By walking the legal decision-maker through the evaluation process and offering the factual basis for opinions *and* the theory or empirical data used to reach the opinions, the mental health professional can more fully present what is really known about gay and lesbian mental health issues. By taking the time to fully explain why a given theory or empirical database has validity *and* is the most appropriate for the interpretation of the "facts" at hand, the mental health professional can better influence the decision-maker to accept the best-informed understanding of gay and lesbian mental health issues that is available.

What follows are some examples of different types of legal proceedings in which a lesbian or gay sexual orientation has been an issue. Examples of some of the questions asked of psychiatrists and other mental health professionals who have testified in these proceedings are given for each type of legal proceeding discussed, along with some of the underlying issues these questions raise.

The information presented here is not the result of a research study or formal analysis. Instead, the information is compiled from my own experiences as a psychiatrist involved in such matters, my discussions with attorneys and other mental health professionals who have been involved in such matters, my review of other cases involving lesbians and gay men, and consultations with individuals whose work has focused on gay and lesbian mental health issues. This discussion is being offered with the hope that it will generate further exploration and discussion, which will in turn result in a more meaningful participation by mental health professionals in legal proceedings in which a lesbian or gay sexual orientation is considered to be an issue.

The overwhelming majority of the cases that form the basis for this discussion involved self-identified lesbians and gay men who were "out" (known to be gay or lesbian) to important homosexual and heterosexual people in their lives. Throughout the rest of this chapter, the reader can assume that I am talking about self-identified, "out" lesbians and gay men, unless otherwise noted. Since I am aware of only a small number of cases that involve self-identified, "out" bisexual or transgender men or women, these cases are not included in this discussion.

As noted earlier, when mental health testimony has been offered in these cases, the testimony has been provided by forensic psychiatrists, treating psychiatrists, and/or a range of other mental health professional forensic experts and therapists. For the rest of this chapter, I will simply refer to "psychiatrists" or "psychiatric opinion," although I will be including the participation of and the opinions rendered by the full range of mental health professionals who might be involved in such matters.

Although the decision-maker in these cases may have been a judge, some type of "hearing officer," or a jury, differences that might exist based on the type of decision-maker are not included in this discussion. Therefore, during the rest of this chapter references to "the court" include any type of trial or legal proceeding in which such matters may be heard and any type of decision-maker who may have been involved.

Child Custody and Visitation Proceedings

The most commonly seen and the most controversial legal proceedings involving lesbians and gays are in the area of family law. Although most of these cases have involved disputes over child custody or visitation, there have also been numerous cases involving foster care placement and adoption.

For the most part, state statutes and the associated guidelines and practices of agencies involved with child welfare matters make no mention of sexual orientation. Those that do mention sexual orientation vary from one state to another, and the statutes, guidelines, and practices across states, or even within a given state, are not always consistent. For example, in New York, gay men and lesbians are guaranteed the same eligibility to become adoptive parents as heterosexuals, whereas in Florida there is still a statutory ban on gay and lesbian adoption (Lilith 2001a). Most states do not expressly prohibit self-identified gay men and lesbians from adopting children, and if the responsible agency simply ignores the sexual orientation of the adoptive parent, the adoptive parent's lesbian or gay sexual orientation may not ever be raised in court. However, in some cases, a court that has been made aware of the lesbian or gay sexual orientation of an adoptive parent has felt the need to determine whether such an adoption would be in the best interests of the child, and in these cases psychiatric opinion has been an important aspect of the case.

Although at present, "second parent adoption" (cases in which a gay or lesbian partner of a legal parent adopts the child of his or her same-gender partner) is permitted in only 21 states (Lilith 2001a), an increasing number of these cases are being presented to the courts. In addition, cases involving reproductive technologies that allow one woman to be a "genetic mother" and her lesbian partner to be the "gestational mother" have presented new challenges to the courts with regard to legal maternity; some courts have found that the child has two legal mothers (Lilith 2001a); but even in cases in which legal maternity was not granted to both lesbian partners, the argument for second-parent adoption is enhanced.

Foster care placement guidelines and practices are usually found not in statutes but in local municipal or other regulations, and therefore guidelines and practices vary considerably from one jurisdiction to another. For example, in cities such as New York and San Francisco, social workers try to match lesbian and gay children with lesbian and gay foster parents, whereas in some other states, it is almost impossible for lesbians and gay men to become foster parents (Lilith 2001a). Although one would expect that foster care placement guidelines and practices would be consistent with state statutes on adoption, this is not always the case. For example, although, as noted earlier, Florida does not permit lesbians or gay men to adopt, they are permitted to become foster parents.

The outcome of child custody or visitation disputes involving a biological parent who is gay or lesbian can certainly be influenced by state statutes, by guidelines and practices governing foster care and adoption that make explicit reference t[...] orientation, and by the presumed "prevailing point of vi[...] influenced them. However, the state statutes that spe[...] govern child custody and visitation matters do not differentiate between heterosexual parents and lesbian or gay parents. More specifically, in all states, all biological parents have certain "inalienable" rights to their children that cannot be taken away from them unless they have a history of and are clearly likely to continue neglecting or abusing their children, or unless a showing of "unfitness" as a parent can be made. Therefore, in disputes between biological parents over the custody of their children, a gay or lesbian parent should be able to obtain custody of the child unless he or she is found to be unfit to parent, or unless the best interest of the child would be better served by placing the child in the custody of the other biological parent. In disputes between a biological parent and a nonbiological parent, a gay or lesbian biological parent should be able to obtain custody of the child unless he or she is found to be unfit to parent or unless the circumstances (i.e., the history of the relationship, or more often the lack of a relationship between the child and the parent) have been so extraordinary as to overcome the legal presumption that favors a biological parent involved in a custody dispute with a nonbiological parent.

Similarly, in all states it is difficult to take away a biological parent's right to visit with his or her child (with the occasional exception of out-of-wedlock fathers). In visitation disputes between a lesbian or gay noncustodial parent and the custodial parent or legal guardian of the child, the lesbian or gay noncustodial parent should be able to continue to have visits with her or his child unless all of the parental rights to the child have been voluntarily given up or involuntarily terminated for cause, or unless visitation is likely to harm the child.

However, in early custody disputes involving a gay or lesbian parent, many courts virtually adopted a "per se rule" that homosexuality disqualified a parent from custody because a homosexual lifestyle was immoral (Eskridge and Hunter 1997). Then, in the 1970s, as courts were pushed to focus specifically on the "best interest of the child," most jurisdictions shifted toward the "nexus approach": the sexual orientation of the parent was no longer "per se" disqualifying, and a denial of custody could be justified only if there was a nexus between the sexual orientation of the parent and harm to the child (Eskridge and Hunter 1997). Although most jurisdictions have now adopted the nexus approach in dealing with custody disputes involving a gay or lesbian parent, some still have presumptions against custody with a gay or lesbian parent, while others have virtually determined that the sexual orientation of the parent is irrelevant (Eskridge and Hunter 1997; Robson 2001). In addition, there is considerable variability in the application of the nexus approach from jurisdiction to jurisdiction; in some jurisdictions there are state statues that require the courts to consider issues that are routinely used to disqualify gay or lesbian parents, such as the "moral fitness" of the parent; in other jurisdictions, judges regularly introduce requirements that ultimately disqualify gay or lesbian parents (Eskridge and Hunter 1997).

Therefore, in most child custody or visitation disputes involving lesbian or gay biological parents, the central question has continued to be whether a lesbian or gay person can be a suitable parent. In a subset of these cases, the question directly or indirectly raised has been whether even allowing a child to visit with a lesbian or gay parent can be so damaging to the child that such contact should be avoided. In other child custody disputes, the gay or lesbian parent's fitness has not been directly challenged, but a central question has been whether the best interest of the child would be better served by placing the child with a heterosexual caregiver.

As previously noted, the state statutes governing child custody and visitation do not specifically mention sexual orientation. However, most state laws that govern child custody and visitation matters permit consideration of a long list of factors that must or may be considered in judging the fitness of parents. All these factors are then open to interpretation by the court that hears a given matter.

Legal precedent is not binding when the issues raised by a given case are new or different from those raised by previous cases. When the court is faced with a gay or lesbian biological parent, the court may find that it must determine whether being gay or lesbian influences the parent's ability to meet existing statutory and nonstatutory standards of fitness, or the court may find that the case raises issues about parental fitness that have not previously been addressed by the state's courts and will therefore have to be addressed as matters of "first impression." The parent's gay or lesbian sexual orientation may therefore be framed as an issue to be resolved as prior, similar cases have been resolved, or it may be said to raise entirely novel issues, or some factor may be said to distinguish the present case from arguably similar prior cases.

In almost all states, parent-centered factors must be considered when judging parental fitness in child custody and visitation matters. These factors include permanence/stability (including employment stability and partner-based stability), moral fitness, mental and physical health, and the ability to give the child the love, affection, and guidance and the spiritual or religious upbringing that he or she requires. State laws also include child-centered factors such as the nature and quality of the bond the child has with each potential custodian or the custodial preference of a child who is considered mature enough to have his or her preference considered by the court.

There have been child custody or visitation disputes involving lesbian or gay biological parents in which the opposing potential custodian asserted that a lesbian or gay parent does not meet statutory standards of parental fitness (Eskridge and Hunter 1997; Robson 2001). For example, it has been directly or indirectly asserted that a lesbian or gay lifestyle is inconsistent with the sense of permanence and stability that a child requires; that being a practicing gay or lesbian person is immoral in and of itself; and that even if being a gay or lesbian person is not technically mentally ill (given the absence of support for this position in DSM-IV) (American Psychiatric Association 1994; see Chapter 4, this volume), it is at least unhealthy. It has also been asserted that a lesbian or gay parent cannot give a child the guidance or spiritual upbringing that a child requires; that such parents will guide a child to become gay, lesbian, or a troubled heterosexual; and that having a gay or lesbian parent is so difficult for a child that it will somehow otherwise damage the child.

Obviously, some of these assertions grow out of a deeply held religious belief or other moral position that being gay or lesbian is wrong. Although legal reliance on religious views has often been questioned, there is probably little that can be done to change the view of those who hold such beliefs and make such assertions. Some of these assertions, particularly those that refer to *the* lesbian or *the* gay lifestyle or point of view, grow out of a stereotypical or even prejudiced view of lesbian or gay persons and a failure to recognize the enormous diversity within the group of people who self-identify as gay or lesbian. Furthermore, some of the other assertions—particularly those that relate to the impact of a gay or lesbian parent on the development of children—are inconsistent with empirical and clinical findings.

Hopefully, psychiatrists and other mental health professionals know that there is no one lesbian or one gay lifestyle or point of view on matters that are important to the parenting of children. Therefore, any lesbian or gay parent must be given the benefit of an individualized assessment as it relates to her or his lifestyle and point of view and how these might or might not impact on the parent's ability to offer the child permanence, stability, a moral environment, guidance, and a generally healthy upbringing. Of course, to perform such an assessment, the psychiatrist must be able to integrate accurate knowledge and a sound understanding of parenting and the needs of developing children with an equally accurate knowledge and a sound understanding of gay and lesbian parents. Similarly, when testifying in child custody and visitation proceedings involving a gay or lesbian parent, psychiatrists must help the court understand that there is enormous diversity within the gay and lesbian community, that the testimony being given is based on an individualized assessment of the particular parent, and that the opinions rendered are supported by the information gathered during the process of the evaluation and by a well-informed body of knowledge that has been used to interpret that information.

In child custody and visitation disputes involving lesbian or gay parents, this "well-informed body of knowledge" must include our best understanding of the potential impact that having a gay or lesbian parent can have on the developing child. It has at times been asserted in such cases that given the difficulties faced by gay and lesbian people in our society, their children are sure to suffer such difficulties too. It has been further asserted that the lives of these children will be more stressful and that, as a result, they will be damaged in some way. In a subset of these cases, it has been specifically asserted that the damage will be of a sexual nature, in that the children will become lesbian or gay or dysfunctional heterosexuals.

Such assertions were made without any real support or with only carefully selected anecdotal support. These assertions also failed to consider whether children might also benefit from having a gay or lesbian parent or this specific lesbian or gay parent and whether children might grow in beneficial ways in response to whatever adversity they might face as a result of having a gay or lesbian parent. However, despite the shortcomings of such assertions, they can be readily heard as valid by a court that already shares such beliefs. Therefore, psychiatrists who testify in such matters must not only present their ultimate findings but also help the court gain a better understanding of the body of knowledge that supports the findings.

There has been considerable social science research on children raised by gay men and lesbians (Ball and Pea 1998; Golombok and Tasker 1996; Patterson and Redding 1996). Most studies have shown that gay and lesbian parents are as likely as heterosexual parents to provide a positive home environment for their children; some studies have suggested that children raised by gay or lesbian parents might even be more likely to develop certain positive attributes, such as tolerance; and most studies have shown that children raised by gay or lesbian parents are no more likely to become homosexual or have sexual difficulties than those raised by heterosexual parents.

Although the results of existing studies of gay and lesbian parenting are enormously helpful, there is clearly still much to be learned about the potential impact of having a gay or lesbian parent on the development of children. Of particular interest is the question of whether being raised by a gay or lesbian parent fosters increased tolerance and other positive attributes. If this ends up being the case, it will become even more reasonable to argue for the inclusion of self-identified gay and lesbian parents in larger studies of parenting, in order to help us find even better ways to raise children who will become adults who are more equipped to struggle with some of the social problems facing our society. Another yet unaddressed and more difficult issue is whether any increased likelihood of homosexuality, or even homosexual exploration, that might be found in children of lesbian or gay parents is actually harmful to children.

Workplace Harassment and Other Discrimination Matters

Gay men and lesbians have brought a range of cases in which they have alleged that they have been harassed, discriminated against, or otherwise victimized at least in part because they are or were perceived to be gay or lesbian. For example, lesbians and gay men have filed cases alleging discrimination based on sexual orientation in the areas of housing and public accommodations, education, disability, and, of course, hate crimes. In the area of employment discrimination, there have been cases related to hiring, retention, and promotion as well as allegations of a "hostile work environment," where gay and lesbian employees are harassed, victimized, or otherwise singled out for differential treatment.

This is an area of the law in which lesbian and gay groups have focused a considerable amount of their attention in an effort to obtain rights and protections that are comparable to those of other historically disenfranchised but now "protected groups." Although efforts to include crimes against gay men and lesbians in "hate crimes" legislation have been the most recently visible of these efforts, there continue to be comparable efforts in the areas of employment, public accommodations, and military participation.

Workplace cases are a good focus for attention, because they raise the full range of issues that can arise in civil matters involving lesbian and gay petitioners.

Title VII of the Civil Rights Act forbids an employer to discriminate against any individual because of race, color, religion, national origin, or sex. Although the types of sex discrimination cases that have been accepted by the courts have expanded over time, the courts have continued to dismiss claims of discrimination based on sexual orientation (Chisholm 2001; Varona and Monks 2000).

Initially, sex discrimination claims focused on the "disparate treatment" of employees who were women; eventually, however, the courts recognized that Title VII also protected men from "disparate treatment" in the workplace (Varona and Monks 2000).

At first, courts dismissed claims of "sexual harassment": "sexual harassment" was viewed as outside the scope of Title VII, and it was also believed that "sexual harassment" was not "because of sex." Eventually, however, "sexual harassment" claims were accepted by the courts if the plaintiff could show that 1) she or he was a member of a protected class, 2) she or he received "unwelcome sexual harassment," 3) the harassment was based on sex, 4) the harassment affected a term or condition of employment, and 5) the employer knew or should have known about the harassment and did not take steps to correct it (Varona and Monks 2000). Although at first the courts limited claims of sexual harassment to cases in which submission to sexual demands was made a condition of employment benefits (i.e., "quid pro quo harassment"), courts later held that Title VII also protected employees from having to work in a "hostile work environment" characterized by such severe or pervasive harassment of a sexual nature that it altered the conditions of employment (Varona and Monks 2000).

Cases involving "same-sex sexual harassment" have had an interesting history in the courts. Although, initially, the courts rejected all such cases, courts now tend to accept cases involving a homosexual harasser. However, when cases have involved harassers who are presumed to be heterosexual, courts have tended to reject these cases on the grounds that they are not "about sex" but about sexual orientation (Chisholm 2001).

Eventually, the courts began to recognize "sex stereotyping" as a form of sex discrimination. Sex stereotyping occurs when an employer discriminates only against men or women who look or act in a way that the employer believes is appropriate only for members of the opposite sex (Varona and Monks 2000). Given that discrimination claims based on sexual orientation are still rejected as uncovered by Title VII, some gays and lesbians have filed claims based on sex stereotyping. In some instances, their claims have been accepted; but in many instances, their claims have been viewed as an attempt to circumvent the lack of Title VII protection based on sexual orientation and have therefore been rejected (Varona and Monks 2000).

The proposed Employment Non-Discrimination Act (ENDA) is patterned after Title VII; it would specifically prohibit employment discrimination based on sexual orientation; however, its terms are not quite as broad as those in Title VII. ENDA has gained broad-based support, and if (when) it is passed, the combination of ENDA and Title VII will effectively close the sexual orientation loophole in federal civil rights legislation (Varona and Monks 2000).

In the absence of federal law prohibiting workplace harassment based on sexual orientation, 11 states and the District of Columbia have enacted laws that protect employees from discrimination based on real or perceived sexual orientation (Chisholm 2001). Through county or city ordinances, a somewhat larger number of gay or lesbian public employees are protected from discrimination based on sexual orientation (Chisholm 2001). However, in many parts of the country, there is still no protection for employees who are discriminated against on the basis of real or perceived sexual orientation. In such instances, claimants must base their claims, at least in part, on the above-described gender-based prohibitions on employment discrimination accepted under Title VII and/or on other equal-protection based claims.

The outcomes of some of the large workplace discrimination and harassment cases involving Title VII–protected groups have had a significant impact on employers. When employers lost those cases and were forced to pay large settlements, they were held liable for not having trained managers, supervisors, and co-workers in diversity issues so that they would not discriminate against or otherwise harass employees in the protected groups. In addition, employers were held liable for not having in place a procedure for employees to file complaints about the discrimination or harassment that they had experienced and/or for not promptly investigating problems that came to their attention and taking remedial action. Therefore, given the outcomes of cases brought to date and the ever-growing diversity of the workforce, employers have come to recognize that it is incumbent on them to provide training on prohibited activities, to have available a procedure for employees to file complaints, and to undertake prompt investigation and remedial action whenever a complaint is filed.

Obviously, in jurisdictions that do not include lesbians and gay men as a protected group, employers generally do not include gay or lesbian issues in company training. However, even in jurisdictions where gay men and lesbians are included as a protected group, many employers either do not realize the need for specific information or may not understand what constitutes harassment of or discrimination against gays and lesbians.

Although most male employees have learned that they should not touch a female supervisee or co-worker in inappropriate ways or make suggestive comments about her body, they do not seem to transfer that knowledge and to grasp that similar behaviors or comments to a gay colleague would be equally unwelcomed and offensive and would therefore be considered harassment by him. Similarly, although most employees know that lewd or degrading comments about the opposite sex are unacceptable in the workplace, they seem unable to recognize that lewd or degrading comments about lesbians or gay men are equally unacceptable. In part, this may be due to unidentified issues of homophobia. For some, gaps in protective laws provide the opportunity to express bias with impunity.

There is even a greater problem recognizing more subtle forms of workplace harassment and discrimination against lesbians and gay men. For example, many employers and co-workers see nothing wrong with telling a gay or lesbian employee that having a picture of a same-sex partner on a desk is a problem for them, even if heterosexual employees have pictures of their partners visible in the office.

Cases claiming "denial of a promotion" or "wrongful discharge" because of sexual orientation are even more complicated, because, as in cases involving other protected groups, employers almost always claim that the failure to promote or the decision to discharge an employee was nondiscriminatory. For example, there is the issue of merit, which could include the person's lack of appropriate education and training, work-related skills, ability to work well with co-workers, ability to supervise other co-workers, or level of experience compared with that of other employees. In addition, promotions based on seniority or other, more political reasons for promoting one employee over another are not at all illegal, and it is often extremely difficult to prove that such reasons are inherently discriminatory.

In all these cases involving lesbian or gay employees, the first issue to prove is that the employer knew that the employee was, in fact, a lesbian or gay or that the employer did, in fact, perceive the employee to be lesbian or gay. When the employee is publicly self-identified as gay or lesbian, this may be somewhat less of an issue. However, when this is not the case and yet the employee believes that the employer either knew that he or she was gay or lesbian or perceived that to be the case, the employee may not be able to get past this first stage of the case.

Then, too, there are cases in which the fact that the employee is lesbian or gay may be only one of the issues that made her or him a focus for harassment or discrimination. There may be compounding issues related to the fact that the employee is a woman, a member of an ethnocultural minority, or a partially disabled person. Psychiatric evaluations performed in such cases become complicated, especially if the employee is uncomfortable about considering how sexual orientation or perceived sexual orientation played a role in the problems at work. Addressing the relevancy of these issues legally may place the lesbian or gay person at risk of greater public exposure. Although sexual orientation may not be the person's issue, public exposure often brings complications in the form of reactions by others. For lesbians and gay men, public revelation of their sexual orientation may expose them to bias and victimization, even by the legal decision-makers charged with their protection.

Furthermore, there is the matter of proving that the workplace environment is hostile toward or that there is discrimination against lesbian or gay employees. This issue must be addressed at the level of the employee's co-workers or supervisor, and it must be shown that the workplace environment is, in fact, hostile or that the employee was, in fact, discriminated against because of sexual orientation. This issue must also be addressed at the level of the company's management, and it must be shown that the company has failed to do what needed to be done to provide a safe work environment or that the company has a pattern of discriminating.

Although it is not the responsibility of a psychiatrist performing an evaluation in such matters to prove that the employee was or was not harassed or discriminated against, the psychiatrist must gain a thorough understanding of what actually happened so as to make an assessment of whether the individual was psychologically harmed as a result of the work experience or whether the individual's problems are a result of non–work-related issues. In cases in which the workplace environment has been hostile, the psychiatrists might also have to help the court understand why certain behaviors were "unwelcomed" by and offensive to a gay or lesbian employee, especially when the decision-maker lacks knowledge about or sensitivity to gay and lesbian issues.

For some lesbian and gay employees, especially those who are not public about their sexuality, "unwelcomed" behaviors may include those that expose their sexual orientation. However, it is important to note that for virtually all lesbian or gay employees, unwelcomed behaviors include a broad range of hostile or otherwise biased comments about lesbian or gay people, sexual innuendos or sexual advances, and false presumptions about how one's sexual orientation affects one's ability to function effectively in the workplace. Gaining an understanding of what behaviors are likely to be "unwelcomed" by and offensive to gay and lesbian employees is critical to understanding workplace harassment cases involving gay and lesbian employees. In addition, including an understanding of what behaviors are likely to be "unwelcomed" by and offensive to gay and lesbian employees with one's broader understanding of unwelcomed and offensive behaviors in the workplace can enrich one's understanding of all workplace harassment cases.

A further issue is whether the employee was psychologically harmed or damaged by whatever happened in the workplace. This is the most important issue that psychiatrists are asked to address in these matters, because the amount of compensation is primarily linked to the extent of the damages and whether the person is likely to ever recover from the damages despite the best therapeutic interventions.

Many petitioners who might not otherwise be inclined to seek treatment for their emotional distress enter treatment. Petitioners who are in treatment are more likely to obtain better compensation for any psychological or emotional harm they might have had as a result of harassment or discrimination in the workplace. This is largely because being in treatment indicates to the court that they have tried to recover from the damages they sustained instead of allowing themselves to just continue to be damaged in an effort to prove or win their case. As a result, the psychiatrist who testifies in these matters may be a forensic psychiatrist or a psychiatrist who is treating the petitioner.

When testifying on psychological or emotional harm, psychiatrists will discover that some courts find it difficult to understand why certain behaviors were so offensive to a gay or lesbian employee and why experiencing such behaviors was so damaging. Therefore, psychiatrists might have to educate the court about a much broader range of lesbian and gay mental health issues. In so doing, they place the workplace experience in context and help the court relate the experiences of the lesbian or gay employee to something in its own experience that can be understood.

Another issue that often arises is the claim by employer defendants that any psychological or emotional difficulties the employee plaintiff might be experiencing are really the result of things outside the workplace. These might include preexisting mental health problems or simultaneously occurring psychosocial stressors. In cases involving lesbian or gay plaintiffs, employer defendants have attempted to shift the blame for a plaintiff's emotional distress to unique or relatively unique extra-work-place stressors—that the employee might have, for example, been voluntarily "coming out" or forced to publicly acknowledge being gay or lesbian, been dealing with the loss of friends as a result of AIDS, or even discovering that he or she is HIV positive.

When the testifying psychiatrist is also the plaintiff's therapist, the psychiatrist is often in the best possible position to discuss the extent to which extra-workplace events have or have not contributed to the plaintiff's psychological or emotional distress. However, when a plaintiff is in treatment and making a claim of psychological or emotional harm, the plaintiff must waive therapist-patient privilege and permit the therapist to disclose all records of the therapy, and this requirement for disclosure continues up until the time of the trial. Knowing that one's treatment records are going to be disclosed, and knowing that once one's therapist is in court he or she may be asked about anything that has come up during the course of treatment, can make a patient reluctant to talk about particularly sensitive issues that the patient does not want exposed. Since the employer defendant might request treatment records even when the plaintiff retains a forensic psychiatrist, the use of a forensic psychiatrist instead of one's treating psychiatrist only partially avoids this problem. Therefore, balancing the requirements for fair adjudication with regard to the patient's mental condition and the patient's treatment needs can become an issue in the therapy that must be directly addressed.

Finally, the litigation process tends to be much more stressful for plaintiffs than they expect it to be. Repeatedly they are professionally and personally attacked at each stage of the process; often they are confronted with things that they really do not want to look at, and they may even be confronted with false accusations. In addition, the plaintiff might be exposed to extremely homophobic insults. This experience can be as damaging or even more damaging than what has already happened to the plaintiff in the workplace, and the risk of further harm is especially great for the plaintiff who did not anticipate how difficult the litigation process could be. Therefore, psychiatrists must anticipate how distressing the litigation process could be for patients involved in these cases and be prepared to provide whatever specific additional assistance or support their patients might require.

Criminal Law and Same-Sex Domestic Violence Cases

In the area of Criminal Law, there have been cases involving gay men or lesbians as the perpetrator of a crime, the victim of a crime, or both the perpetrator and the victim of a crime.

There have been a number of high-profile cases involving a gay predator and multiple victims. In virtually all these cases, the perpetrator's gay sexual orientation was the primary focus of media attention and also dominated the trial, even when it was clear that the perpetrator suffered from major mental health problems. On the other hand, in a number of other cases involving a gay or lesbian perpetrator, the sexual orientation of the perpetrator was never clearly identified or simply positioned as an incidental finding. The mental health issues seen in these cases involving a gay or lesbian perpetrator have been so varied that it is impossible to make generalizations. However, it does appear that, as with cases involving perpetrators from other "minority groups," popular notions about a gay or lesbian perpetrator's sexual orientation (i.e., assumptions or biases about the minority group) can overshadow other issues that might have been more determinative of the person's behavior.

Many of the cases involving lesbian or gay victims have drawn considerable attention, especially when it seemed that the victim became a victim because she or he was, or was at least perceived to be, lesbian or gay. However, although such hate-related crimes seem to horrify everyone who hears about them, in many jurisdictions it has still been difficult to gain the inclusion of crimes against gay men and lesbians in "hate crimes" legislation (Wang 1999; Zwerling 1995). Exactly what this means is difficult to say, but gay and lesbian groups who are working toward the inclusion of these crimes in such legislation believe that although a community might have a very strong reaction to a particularly horrible hate crime perpetrated against an individual lesbian or gay victim, that same community might still view the inclusion of lesbian or gay people in "hate crimes" legislation as endorsing a lifestyle that the community cannot accept. Some social scientists and legal scholars have further argued that "hate crimes" are not simply the result of personal animus, but that they also reflect the larger community's view of the targeted group (Wang 1999).

Another interesting aspect of criminal cases involving lesbian or gay victims has been the defenses put forth by the defendants. For example, some of the heterosexual men who have been perpetrators of violence against gay men have put forth a "homosexual panic" defense, asserting that they experienced an uncontrollable, murderous rage in response to an unwanted sexual advance made by the gay victim. However, in recent years, the "homosexual panic" defense has been much less successful. Although this may be due more to the extent of the acts of violence than to the responsiveness of the finder of fact to arguments against the defense, there have been strong arguments made against such a defense. For example, it has been argued that the concept of "homosexual panic" is controversial, that it has no uniform definition within the behavioral sciences, or that the psychological makeup of the perpetrator does not match any of the definitions of "homosexual panic" that do exist (Suffredini 2001). In addition, it appears that in most cases, the crimes these men have perpetrated against gay men have usually been planned rather than immediate (i.e., "heat of the moment") responses to an encounter with a gay man.

Within the group of cases involving a gay perpetrator and gay victim or a lesbian perpetrator and lesbian victim, domestic violence cases have recently been drawing considerable attention. The New York City Gay and Lesbian Anti-Violence Project (AVP) works with lesbian and gay victims of domestic violence to help them recognize abusive relationships, come forward, and seek help. However, it is actually a broad-spectrum victim services agency that provides counseling to and advocacy for lesbian, gay, transgender, bisexual, and HIV-affected victims of bias and assault. AVP is a member of the National Coalition of Anti-Violence Programs, which is a 26-member national organization.

AVP and the other programs in the coalition are also an important resource for attorneys and mental health professionals who are working on cases involving crimes against gay men and lesbians.

The most comprehensive study of domestic violence within same-sex relationships was conducted by the National Coalition of Anti-Violence Programs. The study found that there was at least some domestic violence in one of four same-sex relationships, which is about the same incidence seen in heterosexual relationships (Knauer 1999). This and other studies have also found the same issues of power and control in same-sex domestic violence, and victims encounter the same forms of abuse and violence, as well as the same cycle of violence, as do their heterosexual counterparts (Jablow 2000; Knauer 1999).

However, victims of same-sex domestic violence can experience some additional forms of abuse on the basis of their sexual orientation. For example, perpetrators often maintain power and control and/or keep the victim from reporting the violence by threatening to reveal the victim's homosexuality or HIV status (Hodges 1999–2000; Knauer 1999; Lilith 2001b). In addition, victims of same-sex domestic violence usually face greater complications in accessing legal protections and safe, sensitive shelter and other services.

Domestic violence cases can be heard in criminal courts, family courts, or domestic relations courts. Therefore, depending on the jurisdiction, domestic violence is not always positioned as a criminal matter; in many instances, it comes up only in the context of a divorce and/or child custody proceeding, and in other instances the victim is simply seeking an "order of protection" or a "restraining order" against the perpetrator.

At the time of this writing, nine states specifically exclude gay or lesbian relationships from their domestic violence statute, by limiting domestic violence to either violence within a male-female relationship or violence within a legal marriage (Hodges 1999-2000). However, since only a few jurisdictions specifically include gay or lesbian relationships in domestic violence statutes, access to legal protection is often limited for victims of same-sex domestic violence (Jablow 2000).

Since police officers are usually the first line of defense in cases of domestic violence, it is critical that they be knowledgeable about and have a clear understanding of domestic violence. There are some jurisdictions with designated domestic violence police officers, and in some of these jurisdictions, such as New York City, training of designated officers includes training about and efforts to develop sensitivity to same-sex domestic violence. However, most frontline police officers do not receive such training about and have not developed any particular sensitivity to same-sex domestic violence.

Similarly, most providers of protection programs and/or clinical services for victims of domestic violence have not yet developed programs or services for victims of same-sex domestic violence. Although in major cities, lesbian and gay groups have begun to provide some services to victims of same-sex domestic violence, there is often still a problem with access to services. In rural areas, services for victims of same-sex domestic violence are often nonexistent.

There is no question that it was women's rights advocates who persuaded the legal profession and the mental health professions that domestic violence is as serious as any other type of violence. However, from both a legal and a mental health perspective, the reasons why it is important to recognize same-sex domestic violence in gay or lesbian relationships are exactly the same reasons why it is important to recognize domestic violence in heterosexual relationships. More specifically, many of the violent behaviors that occur within the context of an intimate relationship may not be taken as seriously if viewed against the backdrop of the full range of violence that occurs within our society. By recognizing that within the context of an intimate relationship there are certain dynamics that do not exist between strangers, it becomes clear that any violence that occurs within an intimate relationship can have a much stronger impact on a person than comparable violence perpetrated by a stranger. These dynamics might include, for example, disruption of trust and the expectation that one is safe within the context of an intimate relationship; a tendency to consider and possibly assume too much responsibility for one's own role in the difficulties in an intimate relationship; and a real or perceived sense of the difficulties involved in getting out of an intimate relationship and away from the violence.

Same-sex domestic violence cases raise other interesting and important mental health issues as well. More specifically, the very existence of same-sex domestic violence, especially in lesbian relationships, appears to raise questions about the well-established paradigm that domestic violence in heterosexual relationships has to do with the power differential between men and women (Knauer 1999). However, those who have focused on same-sex domestic violence have argued that it is actually more accurate to state that the existence of same-sex domestic violence forces us to expand the heterosexual domestic violence paradigm, in that same-sex domestic violence makes it clear that issues other than gender can result in a power differential within an intimate relationship (Hodges 1999–2000; Knauer 1999; Lilith 2001b). These other issues about which there can be a power differential might include, for example, race or ethnicity, socioeconomic status, educational level, religion, immigration status, and health status. Any of these issues can also be used to reinforce victims' perception or experience that they will not receive fair or protective treatment but may in fact be at greater risk away from their abuser. Hopefully, a dialogue that focuses on these and other dynamics used in abusive relationships will become increasingly productive and thereby further improve our ability to understand and to help both victims and perpetrators, regardless of their gender or sexual orientation.

There are also cases that appear to involve mutual violence or a situation in which the distinction between the batterer and the victim is not clear. By definition, an ongoing pattern of mutual violence is something quite different from same-sex domestic violence; it cannot grow out of a power differential in the relationship, and it is also quite different from a situation in which a victim of domestic violence retaliates in fear. However, cases of same-sex domestic violence have often been misperceived as a situation involving mutual violence (Hodges 1999–2000; Lundy 2001), because perpetrators have argued that there has been mutual violence as part of their defense and/or because the court has found it difficult to understand same-sex domestic violence. Cases involving mutual violence raise yet another set of interesting and important mental health issues that need to be further explored and better understood, and such cases must also be more clearly differentiated from cases of same-sex domestic violence.

Obviously, another issue that is central to our understanding of domestic violence is the question of what constitutes a "domestic relationship" in which the dynamics that contribute to domestic violence can occur. This is particularly important with same-sex domestic violence: because lesbians and gay men do not have access to traditional forms of partnering by entering into a marital arrangement, there may be a range of forms of partnering, involving various different living arrangements, different types of reciprocal commitments and agreements, and the like. Therefore, efforts to increase our understanding of the dynamics of domestic violence must include efforts to increase our understanding of the nature and quality of the "domestic relationship" in which same-sex domestic violence may occur. In so doing, we will be better able to educate the court and help the court differentiate between same-sex domestic violence and other forms of violence that lesbians and gay men might encounter.

Immigration and Asylum Cases

The Immigration Act of 1917 specifically excluded gay and lesbian aliens from entering the United States, because of the belief, supported by the psychiatric profession, that homosexuality was a disease (Bennett 1999). This exclusion of gay men and lesbians finally ended in 1990, after Congress recognized that the American Psychiatric Association had removed homosexuality from its list of mental disorders in 1979 (Bennett 1999).

The Refugee Act of 1980 (U.S. Public Law PL 96-212) defined "refugee" as

> any person who is outside any country of such person's nationality or, in the case of a person having no nationality, is outside any country in which such person last habitually resided, and who is unable or unwilling to return to, and is unable or unwill-

ing to avail himself or herself of the protection of, that country because of persecution or a well-founded fear of persecution on account of race, religion, nationality, membership in a particular social group, or political opinion. (U.S. Public Laws 96th Congress 1980)

Then also in 1990, the Board of Immigration Appeals first recognized gays and lesbians as "members of a particular social group" in a case involving the asylum application of Fidel Armando Toboso-Alfonso, who was a gay man from Cuba who feared persecution in his country of origin for being gay (Bennett 1999).

The first time a U.S. immigration court found that gay men and lesbians were "members of a particular social group" was in 1993, when Marcelo Tenorio, a gay man from Brazil, was granted asylum (Bennett 1999). In 1994, then U.S. Attorney General Janet Reno issued a "directive" to U.S. immigration courts, in which she recognized Toboso-Alfonso and Tenorio as precedent-setting cases and indicated that the courts may grant asylum to gays and lesbians on account of their persecution as "members of a particular social group" (Bennett 1999; Soloway 2000–2001). In 2000, the U.S. Court of Appeals for the 9th Circuit further refined this standard in a case involving the asylum application of Geovanni Hernandez-Montiel, who described himself as a homosexual from Mexico with a female sexual identity. In the Hernandez-Montiel case, the 9th Circuit found that in Mexico, homosexual men with female sexual identities were a "particular social group" who were treated differently than homosexual men in general, in that they were particularly targeted for persecution ("Immigration Law—Asylum" *Harvard law Review* 2001).

Historically, there was no specific application deadline for persons seeking asylum in the United States. Then, in 1997, the asylum law was changed for all persons seeking asylum. Specifically, for those who were already in the United States, an application for asylum had to be filed by April 15, 1998, and for all arrivals to the United States after April 15, 1997, an application for asylum must be filed within 1 year after the person arrives in the United States (Soloway 2000–2001). However, the revised law does allow for a waiver of the 1-year application deadline in certain "exceptional" instances. For example, a person might be granted a waiver if a physical or mental health problem "of significant duration" that is related to the failure to file rendered the person unable to file an application within the 1-year deadline, or if there has been a "change in circumstances" that now renders the person at risk of harm upon returning to his or her country of origin. The change in circumstances can be either in the person's home country—usually referring to a change in a regime, in which the new regime would persecute the person, whereas the prior regime would not have—or in the person's personal circumstances—such as religious conversion or recent adoption of unpopular political views that would subject him or her to persecution in the country of origin—rendering the person eligible to apply for asylum, whereas before he or she was not eligible.

Some lesbians and gay men who are seeking asylum in the United States have already sought psychiatric treatment for the difficulties they have experienced as a result of the persecution or fear of persecution they were exposed to in their country of origin. If psychiatric opinion is needed in connection with their application for asylum, their treating psychiatrist is the person most likely to be called. However, many have not sought psychiatric treatment, due to either a lack of insight regarding their need for treatment, a lack of financial resources to pay for treatment (especially since many have fled their countries of origin and come to the United States without papers that would allow them to obtain employment), or an inability to talk about the experiences they have had (which some attorneys have suggested is more common for lesbian and gay asylum seekers than for any other category of "persecuted persons"). Additionally, lesbians and gay men exposed to bias in their country of origin may expect bias from mental health professionals in the United States, especially given that many of those fleeing to the United States are unaware of the fact that homosexuality is no longer considered a mental illness here and that the law barring homosexuals from immigrating to the United States was repealed (Soloway 2000–2001). Therefore, if psychiatric opinion is needed in connection with their application for asylum, they are often referred to a forensic psychiatrist or any other psychiatrist who might be willing to evaluate them and testify on their behalf.

It is not required that an applicant for asylum be suffering from a diagnosable psychiatric disorder in order to be granted asylum. However, psychiatric expert evidence that a person is suffering some type of emotional distress as a result of the persecution or fear of persecution that he or she experienced will help support the person's application, as it will corroborate both the claimed persecution and the basis for the claimed persecution. The applicant must show a "well-founded fear of persecution," by showing both a "subjective fear of persecution" and an "objective fear of persecution" (Bennett 1999). Therefore, applicants and their attorneys seek to submit evidence of the difficulties that lesbians and gay men have in the applicant's country of origin, evidence of any difficulties the applicant might have had, and evidence of physical or psychological injury to the applicant as a result of the difficulties experienced. This body of evidence can be extremely helpful to psychiatrists who perform evaluations in connection with such matters, in that it can help them better understand the case and help them support an opinion that the applicant is not malingering (a matter that is important in virtually all legal proceedings in which psychiatric opinion is offered).

With the 1-year filing requirement instituted in 1997, psychiatrists are also often being asked whether applicants have been suffering from any psychiatric difficulties that rendered them unable to file an application for asylum within the 1-year time frame. In this regard, psychiatric difficulties that impaired the applicant's ability to get out and learn about the asylum option, initiate the application, or follow through with the application process might be relevant. While psychiatric disorders such as posttraumatic stress disorder or major depression could obviously have impaired an applicant's ability to file in a more timely manner, overwhelming fears of the government or fears of repercussion for being openly gay or lesbian might also have interfered with the applicant's ability to file within the required 1-year deadline.

In this regard, it is important to note that many lesbian and gay applicants for asylum based on sexual orientation managed to survive in their country of origin by remaining "closeted," or at least extremely secretive about their sexual orientation. Once such applicants arrive in the United States, many still find it extremely difficult to be more "out" about their sexual orientation, despite the fact that it may appear to them that "out" gay and lesbian Americans are relatively safe and function pretty well. This is a particular problem for gay and lesbian minors who have come to the United States with their parents or other family members, because often their adult family members share the views of those in their country of origin. As long as they are living with or are otherwise dependent on family members, they may find it impossible to "come out" about their sexual orientation. Additionally, many other lesbians and gay men who come to the United States while "closeted" about their sexual orientation typically find themselves dependent on traditional immigrant networks for housing, employment, and also immigration assistance. Often, immigration attorneys are located in particular immigrant or ethnic communities and may also employ individuals from such communities in their offices. Attorney-client privilege as understood in the United States may not be a familiar concept to a newly arrived immigrant who is taken by friends or relatives to an attorney who is a friend of those friends or relatives or a part of the community, especially if the attorney's services are being paid for by those friends or relatives. Therefore, a "closeted" lesbian or gay man may well be reluctant, if not terrified, to reveal her or his sexual orientation to such an attorney.

From both a legal and a psychiatric point of view, the experiences of these previously "closeted" applicants raise two interesting questions. First, given that it is reasonable to argue that an ability to go public with one's sexual orientation is a prerequisite for making an application for asylum based on sexual orientation, can it be argued that an inability to "come out" or go public with one's sexual orientation is an emotional or psychological problem (not necessarily a psychiatric disorder, but an emotional or psychological problem that a psychiatrist can describe) that impaired the applicant's ability to file within the 1-year deadline, thereby allowing the applicant to obtain a waiver of the 1-year deadline once he or she "comes out"? From a legal perspective, although this does not meet the requirement that the person be suffering from "a physical or psychological disability or disease of significant duration," there is the question of whether this might constitute an "exceptional circumstance" warranting an exception. Second, once the applicant has "come out," can this be viewed as a "change in circumstances" (much like changing one's religion) that now makes the applicant at risk of harm if he or she returns home, thereby starting the clock for the 1-year time frame at the time the person "comes out"?

There are asylum cases in which such arguments have been proffered and evidence has been submitted supporting the applicant's assertion that he or she was not "out" before and has now "come out." Although some courts have accepted such arguments, others have not, and courts that have rejected or seriously questioned such arguments have asked applicants why it took them so long to "come out," especially given that they knew that they were gay or lesbian even before they left home.

At present, it is unclear whether or not applicants will continue to be asked why it took them so long to "come out" or why they "came out" now. However, if applicants continue to be confronted with such questions, it is reasonable to suspect that psychiatrists involved in such matters will also be asked to render an opinion on these questions, and it is not at all clear that these are questions that psychiatrists can always render an opinion about.

Certainly there are lesbians and gay men who can identify a particular experience that clearly nudged them "out" or maybe even forced them to "come out." However, for most, "coming out" was more of a gradual process involving a dynamic interplay between self and environment; it was not about making an arbitrary decision, and there may not have been a clear decision point. Although a variety of factors might be identifiable as contributory, no one factor may have been clearly determinative. Although the literature regarding the "coming out" process and complicating factors will certainly be helpful to psychiatrists in addressing this question, it may still take a lot of time to apply what we know about "coming out" to the facts of a particular applicant's life and asylum case.

This issue becomes all the more complicated when one considers the fact that there are persons from countries and cultures that do not even have a name for homosexuality, who may or may not have been consciously aware of their sexual attraction to persons of the same sex when they first came to the United States. In such cases, the possibility of a homosexual way of life may not even have been imagined by the applicant at the time of arrival in the United States, and it may be that exposure to such an option eventually brought homosexual feelings into consciousness.

From a psychiatric point of view, these cases raise other important ethnocultural issues as well. For example, notions of sexual identity and the significance of being labeled as lesbian or gay differ from culture to culture and country to country. In addition, publicly expressing one's sexual identity may be completely foreign to a non-Western lesbian or gay person; at the same time, such a person may have suffered persecution or feared persecution because of a widespread perception that she or he was lesbian or gay. For those who have actually suffered persecution because of a perception that they were lesbian or gay, the persecution might have started in the home when they were still young children, and therefore, as with many abused children, they may find it hard to fully recognize what they experienced as persecution. For those who have not actually been persecuted, a fear of persecution because of being perceived to be lesbian or gay may become all the more real once the person actually publicly identifies as lesbian or gay, even if such public affirmation does not take place until the person arrives in the United States.

Regardless of what position the courts ultimately take on this issue of "coming out," psychiatrists will need to understand the process and find a way to talk about it in a way that is relevant to the questions raised by the courts. However, ultimately, psychiatric opinion in asylum cases will be valid only when psychiatrists can fully consider both the gay and lesbian issues and the many ethnocultural issues raised by these cases.

Conclusion

Even this small sampling of legal proceedings focusing on a lesbian or gay sexual orientation reveals that such cases have raised a wide range of mental health issues. Although offering psychiatric opinion in any of these cases requires an in-depth understanding of what we have already learned about gay and lesbian mental health issues, some of these cases raise other mental health issues that we have only begun to explore.

Each year the number of cases focused on a gay or lesbian sexual orientation continues to grow, and there are also new challenges to existing law or legal precedence. Therefore, it is reasonable to suspect that the laws or legal precedence, at least in certain areas of the law, will continue to evolve, especially in jurisdictions with high concentrations of gay men and lesbians.

Given all of this, our efforts to provide courts with competent expert psychiatric testimony in legal proceedings when lesbian or gay sexual orientation is an issue must be ongoing. We must continue to expand our knowledge about gay and lesbian mental health issues, and we must also keep up with the evolution of the law as it relates to these matters.

Furthermore, there is every reason to suspect that decision-makers' attitudes about and knowledge of gays and lesbians may not evolve as quickly as the law may evolve. Therefore, we will have to continue to be mindful of the importance of educating decision-makers about the psychiatric evaluation process and our knowledge and understanding of the lesbian and gay mental health issues that informs that process.

Finally, there is the role that psychiatry and the other mental health professions play in fostering the evolution of the law or legal precedence. Much of the more discriminatory law in this area is based on what many in our society presume to be true about gay men and lesbians. Therefore, to the extent that our stated knowledge about gay and lesbian mental health issues makes it clear that there is no support found in the behavioral sciences for some of these existing laws, we may be contributing to a change in these laws that would make them more equitable for lesbians and gay men.

References

American Psychiatric Association: Diagnostic and Statistical Manual of Mental Disorders, 4th Edition. Washington, DC, American Psychiatric Association, 1994

Ball CA, Pea JF: Warring with Wardle: morality, social science, and gay and lesbian parents. University of Illinois Law Review 253:287–292, 1998

Bennett AG: The "cure" that harms: sexual orientation–based asylum and the changing definition of persecution. Golden Gate University Law Review 29:279–309, 1999

Chisholm BJ: The (back)door of Oncale v. Sundowner Offshore Services, Inc.: "outing" heterosexuality as a gender-based stereotype. Law and Sexuality 10:239–276, 2001

Eskridge WN, Hunter HD: Families we choose, in Sexuality, Gender, and the Law. Westbury, NY, The Foundation Press, 1997, pp 828–848

Golombok S, Tasker F: Do parents influence the sexual orientation of their children? Findings from a longitudinal study of lesbian families. Dev Psychol 32:3–8, 1996

Hodges KM: Trouble in paradise: barriers to addressing domestic violence in lesbian relationships. Law and Sexuality 9:311–331, 1999–2000

Immigration law—asylum—Ninth Circuit holds that persecuted homosexual Mexican man with a female sexual identity qualifies for asylum under particular social group standard—Hernandez-Montiel v INS 225 F3d 1084 (9th Cir 2000). Harvard Law Review 114:2569–2575, 2001

Jablow PM: Victims of abuse and discrimination: protecting battered homosexual under domestic violence legislation. Hofstra Law Review 28:1095–1145, 2000

Knauer NJ: Same-sex domestic violence: claiming a domestic sphere while risking negative stereotypes. Temple Political and Civil Rights Law Review 8:325–350, 1999

Lilith R: The G.I.F.T. of two biological and legal mothers. American University Journal of Gender, Social Policy and the Law 9:207–242, 2001a

Lilith R: Reconsidering the abuse that dare not speak its name: a criticism of recent legal scholarship regarding same-gender domestic violence, Michigan Journal of Gender and Law 7:181–219, 2001b

Lundy SE: Representing nontraditional families: preventing and protecting against domestic violence, in MCLE Main Handbook. Boston, Massachusetts Continuing Legal Education, Inc, 2001, pp 265–307

Patterson CJ, Redding RE: Lesbian and gay families with children: implications of social science research for policy. Journal of Social Issues 52:29–30, 1996

Robson R: Symposium: "Family" and the political landscape for lesbian, gay, bisexual and transgender people. Albany Law Review 64: 915–948, 2001

Soloway LS: Recent developments in international law: sexual orientation–based asylum claims and federal immigration law. New York University Review of Law and Social Change 26:186–191, 2000–2001

Suffredini KS: Pride and prejudice: the homosexual panic defense. Boston College Third World Law Journal 21:279–314, 2001

U.S. Public Law PL 96-212: Refugee Act of 1980. 96th Congress, 1980

Varona AE, Monks JM: En/gendering equality: seeking relief under Title VII against employment discrimination based on sexual orientation. William & Mary Journal of Women and the Law 7:67–132, 2000

Wang L: The complexities of "hate." Ohio State Law Journal 60:799–900, 1999

Zwerling MS: Legislating against hate in New York: bias crimes and the lesbian and gay community. Touro Law Review 11:529–578, 1995

Chapter 4

Sexual Conversion ("Reparative") Therapies: History and Update

Jack Drescher, M.D.

Many have speculated about the so-called causes of homosexuality. Historically, three types of etiological theories have been presented in the legal, scientific, and medical literature on homosexuality. *Theories of normal variants* define same-sex attraction as a naturally occurring form of sexuality, on a par with heterosexuality. A common normal variant analogy is left-handedness. A second explanation, *theories of pathology*, defines adult homosexuality as a disease or abnormal condition that deviates from a natural, and at times predetermined, heterosexual development. Suggested pathogenic events have included intrauterine hormonal exposure, too much mothering, insufficient fathering, seduction by an older person, a decadent lifestyle, or a spiritual illness. Finally, *theories of immaturity* regard homosexuality as a potentially normal phase—albeit a passing one—to be outgrown on the road to adult heterosexuality (Drescher 1998b).

In 1973, the American Psychiatric Association (APA) endorsed a normal-variant paradigm and removed homosexuality from its list of mental disorders (Bayer 1981). Following the APA's lead, mainstream mental health professions, both in the United States and abroad, adopted the normal-variant paradigm. In 1993, homosexuality was eventually removed from the *International Classification of Diseases* (ICD) as well. Nevertheless, there are some who still maintain that homosexuality represents a form of pathology, immaturity, or both. They continue to advocate for the practice of so-called reparative or sexual conversion therapies that aim to convert a homosexual orientation to a heterosexual one. Some clinicians still offer such treatments, as do religious self-help groups that claim to "heal" homosexuality.

Attempts at converting homosexuality currently occur outside the mainstream of contemporary psychiatric theory and practice (American Psychiatric Association 2000). Therefore, professional efforts to do so raise clinical and ethical issues of concern to all practitioners. To help clinicians better understand the issues involved, this chapter offers a historical overview of clinical attitudes toward homosexuality. It reports on some adverse side effects of sexual conversion treatments that have been either overlooked or ignored in the reparative therapy literature. It then raises important clinical and ethical concerns that emerge when treating patients with same-sex attractions.

Early Modern Theories

Scholars of the modern history of homosexuality often place the beginning of their subject's study in the nineteenth century. In 1864, Karl Ulrichs, a German attorney who could be considered a nineteenth-century equivalent of a gay activist, published *The Riddle of "Man-Manly" Love*. In this treatise, in which he argued against laws criminalizing homosexuality, Ulrichs maintained that some men had a woman's spirit inside them. Drawing, in part, on concepts found in Plato's *Symposium*, he claimed that homosexuality was a normal condition for some people and that such individuals constituted a "third sex." As the term *homosexuality* had not yet been invented, Ulrichs called them "Urnings":

> The Urning is not a man, but rather a kind of feminine being when it concerns not only his entire organism, but also his sexual feelings of love, his entire natural temperament, and his talents. The dominant characteristics are of femininity both in his behavior and his body movements. These are the obvious manifestations of the feminine elements that reside in him. (Ulrichs 1864/1994, p. 36)

It was Ulrichs' contention that homosexuality was normal for members of the third sex.

Several years later, an alternative hypothesis was put forward by Krafft-Ebing in *Psychopathia Sexualis* (1886/1965), a medical compendium of unconventional sexual behaviors. There Krafft-Ebing labeled homosexuality a "degenerative" psychiatric condition. Like many people today, he also believed that individuals are born with a biological predisposition toward homosexuality. In contrast to those who hold the contemporary belief that people are "born gay," however, Krafft-Ebing saw homosexuality not as a normal trait, but as a congenital disease. His medical background notwithstanding, Krafft-Ebing's perspective on homosexuality was firmly grounded in antisexual moral values of the nineteenth century:

> The propagation of the human race is not left to mere accident or the caprices of the individuals, but is guaranteed by the hidden laws of nature which are enforced by a mighty, irresistible impulse. Sensual enjoyment and physical fitness are not the only conditions for the enforcement of these laws, but higher motives and aims, such as the desire to continue the species or the individuality of mental and physical qualities beyond time and space, exert a considerable influence. Man puts himself at once on a level with the beast if he seeks to gratify lust alone, but he elevates his superior position when by curbing the animal desire he combines with the sexual functions ideas of morality, of the sublime, and the beautiful. (Krafft-Ebing 1886/1965, p. 23)

Theories of Immaturity: Freud

A third etiological position to emerge in these early modern debates was advanced by Freud in his *Three Essays on the Theory of Sexuality* (1905/1953). Freud disagreed with Krafft-Ebing's degeneracy theory in general, and with his pathologizing view of homosexuality (or "inversion" as it was then called) in particular:

1. Inversion is found in people who exhibit no other serious deviations from the normal.
2. It is similarly found in people whose efficiency is unimpaired, and who are indeed distinguished by specially high intellectual development and ethical culture.
3. (a) . . . inversion was a frequent phenomenon—one

might almost say an institution charged with important functions—among the peoples of antiquity at the height of their civilization.

(b) It is remarkably widespread among many savage and primitive races, whereas the concept of degeneracy is usually restricted to states of high civilization. (Freud 1905/1953, pp. 138–139)

Freud, also disagreeing with Ulrichs' third-sex theory, claimed that psychoanalysis was "decidedly opposed to any attempt at separating off homosexuals from the rest of mankind as a group of special character" (Freud 1905/1953, p. 145). Freud, instead, contended that homosexuality was a normal part of everybody's development. In his nosology, expressions of adult homosexuality indicated arrested psychosexual development. In 1920, he published a case report of an 18-year-old girl whose parents brought her into treatment after she made a suicidal gesture. The suicide attempt followed her father's disapproval of her refusal to end a relationship with an older woman. Initiating her treatment was problematic:

> . . . parents expect one to cure their nervous and unruly child. By a healthy child they mean one who never causes his parents trouble, and gives them nothing but pleasure. The physician may succeed in curing the child, but after that it goes its own way all the more decidedly, and the parents are now far more dissatisfied than before. In short, it is not a matter of indifference whether someone comes to analysis of his own accord or because he is brought to it—whether it is he himself who desires to be changed, or only his relatives, who love him (or who might be expected to love him). Further unfavorable features in the present case were the facts that the girl was not in any way ill (she did not suffer from anything in herself, nor did she complain of her condition) and that the task to be carried out did not consist in resolving a neurotic conflict but in converting one variety of the genital organization of sexuality into the other. (Freud 1920/1955, pp. 150–151)

Freud's theory of immaturity did not characterize the patient as ill but as having an arrested homosexual "genital organization." He pessimistically noted:

Such an achievement—the removal of genital inversion or homosexuality—is in my experience never an easy matter. . . . In general, to undertake to convert a fully developed homosexual into a heterosexual does not offer much prospect of success than the reverse, except that for good practical reasons the latter is never attempted. (Freud 1920/1955, p. 151)

Freud's theory of immaturity maintained that homosexual instincts were a normal part of every heterosexual's early experience. This theoretical stance allowed for *the possibility* that a gay man or lesbian might sufficiently mature and become a heterosexual, if he or she was sufficiently motivated to do so. One of Freud's final remarks on the subject of sexual conversion therapy is found in his "Letter to an American Mother":

I gather from your letter that your son is a homosexual. I am most impressed by the fact that you do not mention this term yourself in your information about him. May I question you why you avoid it? Homosexuality is assuredly no advantage, but it is nothing to be ashamed of, no vice, no degradation; it cannot be classified as an illness; we consider it to be a variation of the sexual function, produced by a certain arrest of sexual development. Many highly respectable individuals of ancient and modern times have been homosexuals, several of the greatest men among them (Plato, Michelangelo, Leonardo da Vinci, etc.). . . .

By asking me if I can help, you mean, I suppose, if I can abolish homosexuality and make normal heterosexuality take its place. The answer is, in a general way, we cannot promise to achieve it. In a certain number of cases we succeed in developing the blighted germs of heterosexual tendencies which are present in every homosexual, in the majority of cases it is no more possible. (Freud 1935/1960, pp. 423–424)

Theories of Pathology: The Neo-Freudians

After his death, Freud's therapeutic caution was replaced by a more optimistic theory of change. This optimism was to herald reparative therapy's "golden age" (see Drescher 1998a). Psychoanalytic practitioners of the mid–twentieth century based their clinical approaches on the work of Sandor Rado (1940). Rado maintained that Freud's theory of innate bisexuality was in error, that there was no such thing as normal homosexuality, and that heterosexuality was the biological norm:

> The male-female sexual pattern is dictated by anatomy. Almost as fundamental is the fact that by means of the institution of marriage, the male-female sexual pattern is culturally ingrained and perpetuated in every individual from earliest childhood. Homogeneous [i.e., homosexual] pairs satisfy their repudiated yet irresistible male-female desire by means of shared illusions and actual approximations; such is the hold on the individual of a cultural institution based on biological foundations. This mechanism is often deeply buried in the individual's mind under a welter of rationalizations calculated to justify his actual avoidance of the opposite sex. (Rado 1969, p. 212).

Rado believed homosexuality was psychopathological—a phobic avoidance of heterosexuality caused by inadequate, early parenting. His theory had many adherents. Working from a Rado-ite perspective, Bieber et al. (1962) considered "homosexuality to be a pathologic biosocial, psychosexual adaptation consequent to pervasive fears surrounding the expression of heterosexual impulses" (p. 220). Socarides (1968) called homosexuality a "resolution of the separation from the mother by running away from all women" (p. 60). Ovesey (1969) claimed homosexuality was "a deviant form of sexual adaptation into which the patient is forced by the injection of fear into the normal sexual function" (pp. 20–21). These psychoanalytic theories had a significant impact on psychiatric thought in the mid–twentieth century and were part of the rationale for including a diagnosis of "homosexuality" in *Diagnostic and Statistical Manual of Mental Disorders*, 2nd Edition (DSM-II; American Psychiatric Association 1968).

Theories of Normal Variants: The 1973 APA Decision

In the early 1970s, however, the APA began a process that would eventually abandon DSM-II's reliance on the metapsychological formulations of psychoanalysis. Instead, APA was to move toward a diagnostic nosology that used medical and "evidence-based" models. That new manual, *Diagnostic and Statistical Manual of Mental Disorders,* 3rd Edition (DSM-III; American Psychiatric Association 1980), would eventually be published in 1980. Prior to that, however, a series of events led to the 1973 decision by the APA to modify the existing DSM-II and to remove homosexuality per se from the list of mental disorders (Bayer 1981).

The initial impetus for that change came from gay activists, whose protests disrupted the APA's 1970 annual meeting. Those protests eventually led the APA Committee on Nomenclature, which was beginning to formulate DSM-III, to consider whether homosexuality should remain in the diagnostic manual. A subcommittee addressing this issue had the opportunity to study the scientific literature from nonpsychoanalytic sources, a body of work that promoted a normal-variant view of homosexuality. One notable study among this literature was Alfred Kinsey's report that homosexuality was more common in nonpatient populations than was generally believed (Kinsey et al. 1948, 1953). Ford and Beach's (1951) cross-cultural and ethological study confirmed Kinsey's view that homosexuality was not a rare phenomenon. Evelyn Hooker (1957) demonstrated, through impartially interpreted projective tests, that contrary to psychoanalytic theory, nonpatient homosexual men showed no more psychopathology than heterosexual control subjects.

These studies and others led the APA Committee on Nomenclature to conclude that there was greater scientific evidence to support a normal-variant view of homosexuality than there was to support a pathologizing one. They recommended immediately removing homosexuality from DSM-II. Before they could do so, however, the scientific committee was challenged by a petition, organized and signed mostly by psychoanalytic practitioners. The petitioners demanded that the scientific decision be put to a vote by the entire APA membership (Bayer 1981). Despite the analytic protest, the APA membership voted to support the scientific committee, and homosexuality was removed from the diagnostic manual.

In its place, DSM-II carried a new diagnosis of "sexual orientation disturbance"; this diagnosis was based on the concept that homosexuality could be considered an illness if an individual with homosexual feelings found those feelings distressing and wanted to change them. The new diagnosis served the purpose of legitimizing the practice of sexual conversion therapies, even if homosexuality per se was no longer considered an illness. Oddly, the new diagnosis also allowed for the unlikely possibility that a person unhappy with his or her heterosexual orientation might seek treatment to become gay. To reflect the realities of clinical practice, in DSM-III the diagnostic category was renamed "ego dystonic homosexuality." However, since that diagnosis emerged from political compromises made in the 1973 debates—and because it was inconsistent with the evidence-based approach the new diagnostic system was intended to usher in—ego dystonic homosexuality itself was removed from the 1987 revision, DSM-III-R (American Psychiatric Association 1987; see Krajeski 1996). In doing so, the APA fully accepted the normal-variant paradigm in a way that had not been possible 14 years earlier.

A Religious Shift: Tempering Condemnation With Compassion

Paradoxically, as the APA and other scientifically grounded professions adopted a normal-variant paradigm and rejected psychoanalysis' traditional theories of pathology, the latter were being embraced by traditional religious institutions that historically condemned homosexuality:

> The existence of a close link between emotions and sexuality and their interdependence in the wholeness of a personality cannot be denied, even though these two things are diversely understood. In order to talk about a person as mature, *his sexual instinct must have overcome two immature tendencies, narcissism and homosexuality, and must have arrived at heterosexuality.* This is the first step in sexual development, but a second step is also necessary, namely "love" must be seen as a gift and not a form of selfishness. The consequence of this development is sexual conduct on a level that can be properly called "human" . . . Sexual maturity represents a vital step in the attainment of psycho-

logical adulthood. (National Conference of Catholic Bishops 1982, p. 167; emphasis added)

Psychoanalytic theories of immaturity and pathology—now discredited in the mental health mainstream—became increasingly important to many religious denominations that were struggling to temper their compassion for homosexual individuals with their historic, antihomosexual traditions of outright condemnation (Coleman 1995; Harvey 1987). This process led some religions to adopt a modern moral imperative to "love the sinner but hate the sin." From this contemporary religious perspective, gay men and lesbians do not have to be automatically expelled or shunned by their community of faith. Instead, they are embraced if they will renounce their homosexuality and seek to "cure" it. This changing environment led to a growing movement of religiously based self-help groups for individuals who refer to themselves as "ex-gay" and who believe that

> [h]omosexuality is not the word of God—nor is it usually a person's choice. Homosexuality is an aspect of underdeveloped sexuality resulting from no one simple factor. Homosexuality of itself is not a sin—it does not make a person sick or perverse. Homosexual acts, however, are wrong—and do not lead a person to deeper life in Jesus Christ. . . . We are not the cause of our loved one's homosexuality but we are responsible to help them live and grow as Catholic Christians. Reparative growth to a fuller possession of heterosexuality is possible for those so motivated.[1]

The ex-gay movement, primarily comprising religious lay people struggling against their homosexual feeling, receives varying degrees of support from organized religious and political institutions (Dreyfuss 1999). However, some mental health practitioners subscribe to this religious perspective as well (Moberly 1983; Nicolosi 1991; van den Aardweg 1997). Elizabeth Moberly (1983), who coined the term "reparative therapy," takes a clinical stance whose foundation is built on scripture rather than science:

---

[1]Quoted from an undated flyer published by an ex-gay ministry called Courage and En-Courage.

Traditionally, the Christian faith has regarded homosexual activity as inappropriate, as contrary to the will and purposes of God for mankind . . . it seems to the present writer that one may not avoid the conclusion that homosexual acts are always condemned and never approved. *The need for reassessment is not to be found at this point.* (p. 27; emphasis added)

Moberly's approach seamlessly combines psychoanalytic theories with her religious beliefs. She calls homosexuality an illness caused by "some deficit in the relationship with the parent of the same sex. . . . Any incident that happens to place a particular strain on the relationship between the child and the parent of the same sex is potentially causative" (pp. 2–3). Unlike Freud, she sees homosexuality's very existence as implying illness, regardless of the actual functioning of the homosexual individual:

The common factor in every case [of homosexuality] is disruption in the attachment to the parent of the same sex, however it may have been caused. Whatever the particular incident may be, it is something that has been experienced as hurtful by the child, whether or not intended as hurtful by the parent. . . . it must be emphasized that this relational defect may not be evident, or not more than partially evident to appearances. At the conscious level an adjustment may be made that leaves few or even no signs of disturbance. The family relationships of a homosexual may in a number of instances seem to be good, indeed, in such cases they are good at a certain level. This is not an objection to the present hypothesis, since what we are speaking of is intrapsychic damage at a deep level, much of which may not be overt or conscious. Similarly, it may not always be readily evident what led to the deficit in the first place. The cause may not be readily recognized, or recognized for what it is. (Moberly 1983, p. 4)

The techniques offered by religious reparative therapies require patients to submit to religious teachings that condemn homosexuality—teachings that are shared and repeated by the therapist or fellow, ex-gay group members. This faith-healing approach may inhibit overt behavioral expressions of homosexual activity. Since "reparative therapy is not a 'cure' in the sense of erasing all homosexual feelings," (Nicolosi 1991, p. xviii), individuals who cannot change are encouraged to inhibit any homosexual behaviors and to remain celibate.

The Clinical Debate's Political Dimension: The Culture Wars

It is noteworthy that the APA's 1973 decision deprived religious, political, governmental, military, media, and educational institutions of any medical or scientific rationalization for discrimination. Without that cover, particularly in the last decade, a historically unprecedented social acceptance of openly gay men and women ensued. With gay men and lesbians no longer considered ill and in need of treatment, society had to come to moral and legal terms with how gay people were to openly live their lives. However, it remained to be seen under what conditions they could love, work, and create new families. Today these moral and legal debates have come to be known as the "culture wars" (Dreyfuss 1999).

In parallel with the 1973 APA debate, the opposing sides in today's culture wars argue from the belief that 1) homosexuality is normal and acceptable or 2) homosexuality is neither normal nor acceptable. The former position is what I call the *normal/identity model*. In the tradition of Kinsey, Ford and Beach, and Hooker, its underlying proposition is that homosexuality is a normal variation of human expression. This position rejects historical cultural beliefs that homosexuality represents either illness or immorality. The acceptance of one's normal homosexual orientation is regarded as a distinguishing feature of a gay or lesbian identity. This position further defines individuals with a gay or lesbian identity as members of a sexual minority. This position holds that, as members of a minority, gay men and lesbians need protection from discrimination by the heterosexual majority.

The opposing position in this debate adheres to what I call the *illness/behavior model*. One of its central tenets is a forceful rejection of the normal/identity model. This position regards any open expressions of homosexuality as pathognomonic of psychiatric illness, a moral failing, or both. A normal identity cannot be created from illness or sin, nor does it provide the basis for defining membership in a (sexual) minority group. Thus, those who engage in homosexual behavior are not akin to racial, ethnic, or religious minorities.

After 1973, the illness/behavior model was gradually marginalized from the mental health mainstream. However, it was born again elsewhere as the clinical argument that homosexuality is an illness meshed seamlessly with a social-conservative, political message: homosexuality is a "behavior," not an "identity." If homosexual behavior can be changed in just one person, then gay people cannot be considered a minority entitled to legislative protections. For example, this interweaving of clinical theory and conservative politics led *The Wall Street Journal* to run an op-ed piece written by sexual conversion therapists arguing that individuals unhappy about their homosexual feelings should have the right to seek treatment for change (Socarides et al. 1997). The aggressive marketing of heterosexuality (see Drescher 1999) eventually reached its peak in a series of expensive, full-page newspaper advertisements that trumpeted successful sexual orientation conversions (Dreyfuss 1999).

Caveat Emptor: Conversion Therapy's Failures and Risks

What is not said in the fine print when advertisers claim conversion therapy success? Bieber et al. (1962) claimed a 27% conversion rate of homosexual patients into heterosexual ones through traditional psychoanalytic methods. Those results have been seriously questioned (Moor 2001; Tripp 1975). Furthermore, little mention is made of the 73% of patients who did not change. In a chapter titled "The Results of Treatment," the authors of the Bieber study focused primarily on how to distinguish those patients who were reported to have changed from those who did not. No harmful effects of the treatment were reported. Socarides (1995), commenting on 10 years of treating homosexual patients, claims a psychoanalytic conversion rate of 35% (p. 102). He, too, does not mention any untoward effects of treatment on the other 65% of his patients, although he does describe some of them:

Some simply had to move away because their jobs took them elsewhere. Some ended treatment because of their fears that emerged from their unconscious—fears that were responsible for their homosexual needs, and which they didn't have the courage to face, and try to conquer. Some may have simply been reluctant to change their lifestyles. This is true of some alcoholics. If they give up drinking, they have to start looking for a whole new set of friends. (Socarides 1995, p. 102)

Socarides' comments exemplify a consistently narrow focus in this literature, which reports therapeutic successes while making no mention of any harmful side effects. Discussions of treatment success and failure tend to focus on the issue of patient motivation, which appears to be the only selection criterion used to choose patients. Ovesey (1969)—who asserts that "those who seek treatment are candidates for treatment; those who don't are not" (p. 118)—makes explicit the reparative therapist's belief that anyone who wishes to change his or her homosexuality should be given the opportunity to do so. A corollary, implicit belief is that any price is worth paying to become a heterosexual. Reparative therapists' idealization of heterosexuality may explain why their literature is silent about any untoward effects of seeking to change one's sexual orientation.

Instead, reports of the adverse effects of sexual conversion therapies have come from other sources. These include a growing number of memoirs and self-reports by gay people who have seen therapists in efforts to change their sexual orientation (Carrol 1997; Duberman 1991; Isay 1996; White 1994). Mel White, a former Jerry Falwell speechwriter, offers a perspective that is rarely reported in the reparative therapy literature:

I read and memorized biblical texts on faith. I fasted and prayed for healing. I believed that God had "healed me" or was "in the process of healing me." But over the long haul, my sexual orientation didn't change. My natural attraction to men never lessened. My need for a long-term, loving relationship with another gay man just increased with every prayer.

After months of trying, my psychiatrist implied that I wasn't really cooperating with the Spirit of God. "He is trying to heal you," the doctor said, "but you are hanging on to the old man and not reaching out to the new." After that, my guilt and fear just escalated.

In fact, the doctor was wrong. He had promised me that if I had enough faith, God would completely change my sexual orientation. I was clinging to that promise like a rock climber clings to the face of a cliff. You can imagine how confused and guilt-ridden I became when my homosexuality stayed firmly in place and the new heterosexual man I hoped to become continued to elude me. (White 1994, p. 107)

Reparative therapists claim a patient's lack of motivation is the primary obstacle to change. However, the assumption that motivation is the primary transformative factor usually leads to patient-blaming when the patient does not convert (Drescher 1997). White, for example, felt blamed by his therapist for the treatment's failure, a failure that exacerbated his own feelings of anxiety, impotence, guilt, and depression. Other therapists, in attempts to effect a sexual orientation conversion, have told their gay patients to either end their same-sex relationships or end therapy (Duberman 1991). Others have encouraged their patients to marry and start families, which later dissolved when the unchanged patient "came out" as gay (Isay 1996; White 1994). The psychological consequences of such treatment outcomes—for unchanged patients, their abandoned same-sex partners, and their shattered heterosexual families—is not commonly reported in the reparative therapy literature, if at all. Yet sexual conversion therapists ignore these troubling anecdotal reports and instead shift the focus to their repeated political cum clinical message, which is that any individual seeking to change his or her homosexual orientation should be provided access to such treatment (Yarhouse 1998).

Anecdotal reports are now beginning to be studied in a more systematic way. In one recent study, Schroeder and Shidlo (2001) interviewed 150 individuals who had unsuccessful conversion therapies. On the basis of their subjects' responses, the authors identified numerous ethical violations by practitioners in the area of informed consent, confidentiality, coercion, pretermination counseling, and provision of referrals after treatment failure. As in the following example from the reparative therapy literature,

Schroeder and Shidlo found that these practitioners are cavalierly dismissive, if not contemptuous, of the normal/identity model:

> Scientific evidence has confirmed that genetic and hormonal factors do not seem to play a determining role in homosexuality. However there continue to be attempts to prove that genetics rather than family factors determines homosexuality. These continuing efforts reflect the persistence of gay advocates to formulate a means by which homosexual behavior may be viewed as normal.
>
> The question of a biological basis for homosexuality has also been reopened due to pressure for minority-rights status for homosexuals. Justification for this special civil-rights status would be supported if scientific evidence could be found that homosexuality is inborn. Opponents of this special-rights status, on the other hand, view homosexuality as an acquired behavior. Gays usually strongly believe they were "born this way." The more deeply identified a person is with his sexual orientation, the more he prefers to believe it was prenatally determined (Nicolosi 1991, pp. 87–88)

Schroeder and Shidlo found that, in an ethically questionable approach to informed consent regarding the current state of scientific knowledge, these therapists often tell potential patients that the positions of both the American Psychiatric Association and the American Psychological Association are based on political pressure from the gay community and not on empirical research. Other therapists referred to the 1973 decision as "secular information that should not have bearing on religion-based psychotherapy." Many of the study's subjects were told by their therapists that all gay people live unhappy lives and that gay relationships are undesirable, unhealthy, and unhappy. The reparative therapy literature is rife with such claims:

> Gay couples are characteristically brief and very volatile, with much fighting, arguing, making-up again, and continual disappointments. They may take the form of intense romances, where the attraction remains primarily sexual, characterized by infatuation and never evolving into mature love; or else they settle into long-term friendships while maintaining outside affairs. Research, however, reveals that they almost never possess the mature elements of quiet consistency, trust, mutual depen-

dency, and sexual fidelity characteristic of highly functioning heterosexual marriages. (Nicolosi 1991, p. 110)

Other troubling ethical concerns raised by Schroeder and Shidlo's study are found in the accounts of former students of religious universities. Many of them said they were coerced into treatment by their schools. They reported that their confidentiality was routinely breached by therapists or counselors who reported a patient–client's ongoing homosexual activity to school officials or even to family members without prior consent. Patients who eventually decided they were gay or lesbian and wished to leave treatment were pressured by their therapists to stay. Many therapists would not accept a patient's decision to accept his or her homosexual feelings and adopt a gay or lesbian identity. If they did leave, patients were not provided with adequate referrals to therapists who might be more supportive and helpful in integrating a gay identity. This is a troubling finding in light of Haldeman's (2001) report of his work with gay men who had left sexual conversion therapies. He found many suffered from intimacy avoidance and sexual dysfunction, as well as depression and guilt related to losing the support of their community of faith.

In light of growing concern about these adverse effects, the American Psychiatric Association's Board of Trustees issued a 1998 position statement saying "the APA opposes any psychiatric treatment, such as 'reparative' or conversion therapy, which is based upon the assumption that homosexuality per se is a mental disorder or based upon the a priori assumption that a patient should change his/her sexual homosexual orientation. In doing so, the APA joined other professional organizations that either oppose or are critical of reparative therapies." It is the APA's position that

[t]he potential risks of "reparative therapy" are great and include depression, anxiety, and self-destructive behavior, since therapist alignment with societal prejudices against homosexuality may reinforce self-hatred already experienced by the patient. Many patients who have undergone "reparative therapy" relate that they were inaccurately told that homosexuals are

lonely, unhappy individuals who never achieve acceptance or satisfaction. The possibility that the person might achieve happiness and satisfying interpersonal relationships as a gay man or lesbian are not presented, nor are alternative approaches to dealing with the effects of societal stigmatization discussed. (American Psychiatric Association 1998/1999)

In 2000, in a follow-up position statement by its Commission on Psychotherapy by Psychiatrists (COPP), the APA expanded and elaborated on the Board of Trustees' earlier statement in order to further address public and professional concerns about therapies designed to change a patient's sexual orientation or sexual identity. COPP recommended that "ethical practitioners refrain from attempts to change individuals sexual orientation" and urged the APA "to encourage and support research in the NIMH and the academic research community to further determine reparative therapies risks versus its benefits." Insofar as inadequately studied reports of "cures" are counterbalanced by claims of psychological harm, "COPP recommends that ethical practitioners refrain from attempts to change individuals' sexual orientation, keeping in mind the medical dictum to first, do no harm" (American Psychiatric Association 2000).

Conclusion

In calling for a moratorium on sexual conversion treatments, organized psychiatry has acted forcefully to protect patients who may be harmed by those procedures. Furthermore, in calling for further research on the risks versus benefits of such treatments, the APA recognizes that some individuals may still wish to change their sexual orientation for religious or other reasons. Even if homosexuality per se is not a mental disorder, psychiatry and other mental health professions must find a way to help individuals who wish to rid themselves of same-sex feelings. However, this cannot and should not be done by accommodating religious requests to redefine homosexuality as an illness.

If psychiatry is to play a role in assisting such patients, perhaps the field of plastic surgery might serve as a model: Plastic surgeons devote much time, energy, and resources to treating non-pathological but socially stigmatized physical conditions. Plastic surgeons, however, employ standards of care that are not matched by those of sexual conversion therapists. For example, in the past, medical reparative therapists failed to develop scientifically and clinically sound selection criteria for patients. As one psychiatrist put it, ". . . those who seek treatment are candidates for treatment; those who don't are not" (Ovesey 1969, p. 118).

It remains uncertain if more exacting standards of care can be developed by today's sexual conversion therapists. After the mental health mainstream endorsed a normal-variant model and the social acceptance of homosexuality increased, the professional training, credentials, and standing of sexual conversion therapists inversely diminished. A field once dominated by medically trained practitioners (Bieber et al. 1962) is now primarily the province of master's-level clinicians, pastoral counselors, and self-help groups. Many of today's reparative therapists work within a faith-healing model. Therefore, it remains to be seen whether they can successfully develop scientific and clinical selection criteria to distinguish individuals who have a reasonable prospect of changing their sexual orientation from those who may be harmed by sexual conversion treatments. Until reparative therapists are able to generate more rigorous selection standards, the dictum to "first do no harm" serves as an appropriate reminder from those concerned about the well-being and the quality of care for all patients, regardless of their eventual sexual orientation.

References

American Psychiatric Association: Diagnostic and Statistical Manual of Mental Disorders, 2nd Edition. Washington, DC, American Psychiatric Association, 1968

American Psychiatric Association: Diagnostic and Statistical Manual of Mental Disorders, 3rd Edition. Washington, DC, American Psychiatric Association, 1980

American Psychiatric Association: Diagnostic and Statistical Manual of Mental Disorders, 3rd Edition, Revised. Washington, DC, American Psychiatric Association, 1987

American Psychiatric Association: Position statement on psychiatric treatment and sexual orientation (1998). Am J Psychiatry 156:1131, 1999

American Psychiatric Association, Commission on Psychotherapy by Psychiatrists (COPP): Position statement on therapies focused on attempts to change sexual orientation (reparative or conversion therapies). Am J Psychiatry 157:1719–1721, 2000

Bayer R: Homosexuality and American Psychiatry: The Politics of Diagnosis. New York, Basic Books, 1981

Bieber I, Dain H, Dince P, et al: Homosexuality: A Psychoanalytic Study. New York, Basic Books, 1962

Carrol W: On being gay and an American Baptist minister. The InSpiriter, Spring 1997, pp 6–7, 11

Coleman G: Homosexuality: Catholic Teaching and Pastoral Practice. Mahwah, NJ, Paulist Press, 1995

Drescher J: What needs changing? Some questions raised by reparative therapy practices. New York State Psychiatric Society Bulletin 40(1): 8–10, 1997

Drescher J: I'm your handyman: a history of reparative therapies. J Homosex 36(1):19–42, 1998a

Drescher J: Psychoanalytic Therapy and the Gay Man. Hillsdale, NJ, Analytic Press, 1998b

Drescher J: The marketing of heterosexuality. Newsletter of the Association of Gay and Lesbian Psychiatrists 25(2):10, 17, 1999

Dreyfuss R: The holy war on gays. Rolling Stone, March 18, 1999, pp 38–41

Duberman M: Cures: A Gay Man's Odyssey. New York, Dutton, 1991

Ford C, Beach F: Patterns of Sexual Behavior. New York, Harper, 1951

Freud S: Three essays on the theory of sexuality (1905), in Standard Edition of the Complete Psychological Works of Sigmund Freud, Vol 7. Translated and edited by Strachey J. London, Hogarth Press, 1953, pp 123–246

Freud S: The psychogenesis of a case of homosexuality in a woman (1920), in Standard Edition of the Complete Psychological Works of Sigmund Freud, Vol 18. Translated and edited by Strachey J. London, Hogarth Press, 1955, pp 145–172

Freud S: Anonymous [Letter to an American mother] (1935), in The Letters of Sigmund Freud. Edited by Freud E. New York, Basic Books, 1960, pp 423–424

Haldeman D: Therapeutic antidotes: helping gay and bisexual men recover from conversion therapies. Journal of Gay and Lesbian Psychotherapy. 5(3–4):119–132, 2001

Harvey J: The Homosexual Person: New Thinking in Pastoral Care. San Francisco, CA, Ignatius, 1987

Hooker E: The adjustment of the male overt homosexual. Journal of Projective Techniques 21:18–31, 1957

Isay R: Becoming Gay: The Journey to Self-Acceptance. New York, Pantheon, 1996

Kinsey A, Pomeroy W, Martin C: Sexual Behavior in the Human Male. Philadelphia, PA, WB Saunders, 1948

Kinsey A, Pomeroy W, Martin C, et al: Sexual Behavior in the Human Female. Philadelphia, PA, WB Saunders, 1953

Krafft-Ebing R: Psychopathia Sexualis (1886). Translated by Wedeck H. New York, Putnam, 1965

Krajeski J: Homosexuality and the mental health professions, in Textbook of Homosexuality and Mental Health. Edited by Cabaj RP, Stein TS. Washington, DC, American Psychiatric Press, 1996, pp 17–31

Moberly E: Homosexuality: A New Christian Ethic. Cambridge, UK, James Clarke, 1983

Moor P: The view from Irving Bieber's couch: "Heads I win, tails you lose." Journal of Gay and Lesbian Psychotherapy 5(3–4):25–36, 2001

National Conference of Catholic Bishops: Norms for Priestly Formation. Washington, DC, United States Catholic Conference, 1982

Nicolosi J: Reparative Therapy of Male Homosexuality: A New Clinical Approach. Northvale, NJ, Jason Aronson, 1991

Ovesey L: Homosexuality and Pseudohomosexuality. New York, Science House, 1969

Rado S: A critical examination of the concept of bisexuality. Psychosom Med 2:459–467, 1940

Rado S: Adaptational Psychodynamics: Motivation and Control. New York, Science House, 1969

Schroeder M, Shidlo A: Ethical issues in sexual orientation conversion therapies: an empirical study of consumers. Journal of Gay and Lesbian Psychotherapy 5(3–4):133–168, 2001

Socarides C: The Overt Homosexual. New York, Grune & Stratton, 1968

Socarides C: Homosexuality: A Freedom Too Far. Phoenix, AZ, Adam Margrave Books, 1995

Socarides C, Kaufman B, Nicolosi J, et al: Don't forsake homosexuals who want help. The Wall Street Journal, January 9, 1997

Tripp CA: The Homosexual Matrix. New York, Meridian, 1975

Ulrichs K: The Riddle of "Man-Manly" Love (1864). Translated by Lombardi-Nash M. Buffalo, NY, Prometheus Books, 1994

van den Aardweg G: The Battle for Normality: A Guide for (Self-) Therapy for Homosexuality. San Francisco, CA, Ignatius Press, 1997

White M: Stranger at the Gate: To Be Gay and Christian in America. New York, Simon & Schuster, 1994

Yarhouse M: When clients seek treatment for same-sex attraction: ethical issues in the "Right to Choose" debate. Psychotherapy: Theory, Research, Practice, Training 35(2):248–259, 1998

Chapter 5

Transgender Mental Health

The Intersection of Race, Sexual Orientation, and Gender Identity

Donald E. Tarver II, M.D.

In the 18th century, racism in the United States of America permeated medical and psychiatric classification. The adaptive, normative coping traits and behaviors of black slaves were medically diagnosed as psychiatric disorders. The attempt to escape from slavery and the depression of being enslaved were entered into medical nomenclature as if these were psychopathological conditions.

Until 1973, homosexuality was also considered to be an official psychiatric disorder. In some communities in the United States today, social and psychological conceptions of transgender identity are progressing toward a normative model. Many cultures of the past and present world have long considered transgenderism to be native and essential within their concepts of sexual diversity and constructed gender roles.

The trend toward reevaluation and depathologizing of transgender identity is also happening in contemporary psychiatric practice as well. Accordingly, gender identity disorder should follow the sequential declassification of its racist predecessors and of the declassification of homosexuality as a mental disorder by the American Psychiatric Association between 1973 and 1987 (American Psychiatric Association 1987).

In this chapter, I examine the public and professional evolution of thinking toward the U.S. African race (a.k.a., African American or Black American) and toward sexual orientation (Davison 1976) with regard to the emergent reevaluation of the psychiatric diagnosis and treatment of gender identity disorder.

Psychiatric Diagnosis and U.S. Africans

There are historical examples of classification of members of a socially stigmatized population as inherently mentally disordered on the basis of a socially influenced psychiatric construction. U.S. African slaves who sought repeatedly to escape were at one time diagnosed with "Drapetomania, or the Disease Causing Negroes to Run Away" (De Bow's Review 1851/1967). A religious belief asserting that "the position that we learn from the Scriptures [that] he [the Negro slave] was intended to occupy, that is, the position of submission" was used to justify the diagnosis by the physician and author, Dr. Cartwright. Dr. Cartwright also established the medical diagnosis of "Dysaesthesia Aethiopica—A Disease Peculiar to Negroes—Called by Overseers, 'Rascality.'" This "species of mental disease," Dysaesthesia Aethiopica, was considered by Dr. Cartwright as an incurable and universal mental disorder of free Negroes and poorly governed slaves. Dysaesthesia Aethiopica was socially constructed as attributable to "the natural offspring of negro [sic] liberty."

These diagnostic terms are viewed as antiquated and offensive by the social standards of today. Yet only 137 years—as few as six family generations—have passed since the federal order mandating the emancipation of slaves reached Texas, the westernmost slaveholding state. Such dehumanizing attitudes and racism persist today and continue to have a pervasive negative biopsychosocial impact on U.S. Africans (McLeod and Kessler 1990). Although no longer subject to a psychiatric classification based on the social framework of slavery, U.S. Africans have been repeatedly shown in modern studies to encounter a disproportionate incidence of psychiatric misdiagnosis and, as a result, improper psychiatric treatment (Adebimpe 1994). The most common true mental health issues for U.S. Africans—depression, anxiety disorders, and mental disorders due to medical conditions—parallel the issues with which gay, lesbian, bisexual, and transgender persons who seek assistance present. These issues include the "dysphoria" of experiencing misunderstanding and traumatic mistreatment by others; overt and covert discrimination in access to health care, housing, and employment resources; and the experience of being scorned and marginalized by a majority population (Priest 1991).

Differentiating Gender From Sexual Orientation

Sexual orientation, in contrast to gender identity, reflects the *interpersonal* sexual attraction of one person toward another person. *Homosexuality* is a clinical term referring to same-sex attraction. Sexual orientation applies to transgender persons *according to their gender of psychological identity*, not to their gender as assigned at birth. For example, a transgender woman, identified as an anatomical male at birth but now identifying and living as a woman, may be described as homosexual or lesbian if she is primarily sexually attracted to other women. By contrast, a transgender woman who is primarily attracted to men may be considered heterosexual.

Many transgender persons and persons who are not of transgender identity, male and female, have varying degrees of sexual attraction to both males and females and are therefore bisexual. *Heterosexuality* refers to attraction of one person to another of the "opposite" gender or sex. *Bisexuality* identifies persons who are attracted to women and men, to varying degrees. *Pansexuality* or *polysexuality* represents the broader sense attraction to persons of diverse gender attributes. For example, a pansexual woman may be attracted at times to some biological women, to biological men, and to some transgender women (biological males living as women, often with a female psychological, hormonal, and surgical gender).

Declassifying Homosexuality

In the 1930s, a Committee for the Study of Sex Variants (The Kinsey Institute for Research in Sex, Gender and Reproduction, New

York, New York) was formed to psychologically and physically examine men and women who volunteered to further the understanding of homosexual and transgender identities. The subjects included men and women with same-sex attraction (homosexual), as well as men who were born and raised as female children until, as adults, they adopted full-time a male gender identity. Although some of these subjects were lesbians inclined to cross-dress and to cross-live in order to cope with social prohibition of woman-to-woman sexual relationships, it is likely that at least some male-identified subjects who were biologically born as female had come to realize a psychological transgender male identity. In fact, the first recorded sex reassignment (i.e., sex change, gender reassignment, or gender confirmation) surgery was performed as early as 1930 for Lili Elbe, a German male-to-female transgender woman.

Among homosexual and heterosexual women and men, cross-gender behavior is also commonly undertaken for theatrical performance, employment as male or female impersonators (sometimes self-identified as "drag kings" or "drag queens"), avoidance of gender-based sex roles such as military induction, or access to gender-restricted occupational roles. One historical example of occupational transgenderism is the report that Deborah Gannet, a U.S. African woman, cross-dressed to serve as a male soldier in the Massachusetts 4th Regiment in 1784 (Israel and Tarver 1997).

Social Norms of Gender

Transgender or cross-gender dress and behavior have historical and contemporary precedents in many cultures. Many deities of antiquity had unequivocal characteristics of both male and female sexes. Cave paintings of such deities, perhaps representing true biologically intersex persons, have been found in Cro-Magnon dwellings. The Egyptian pharaoh Hapchetsut ruled from 1504 to 1484 B.C. as a biological woman cross-dressed as a man. Sometimes viewed as homosexual, Native American "two spirit people" are biological males sanctioned to engage in the tribal work usually performed exclusively by women. In India, there is a long and enduring tradition of boys leaving their families to become members of the Hijra, spiritually anointed eunuchs, ritually or surgically castrated, who dress and live as women to fulfill well-established community functions within Indian society.

In San Francisco, progressive social attitudes have resulted in a city ordinance broadly prohibiting discrimination based on gender identity. Transgender persons are granted the legal right to self-identify their gender based on genetics, biology, anatomy, hormones, spirituality, culture, politics, or psychology. The identification of gender entitles the transgender person to access the housing, health care, educational, and occupational services suitable to her or his gender identity. The legal and psychological power is intended to shift from a controlling observer to the transgender person. Certainly not perfect in its implementation or enforcement, this local ordinance supports the rights of the transgender individual to equal protection under law and to full social integration. Under the terms of this ordinance, it is no longer a legal option for psychiatrists and other authority figures to regard a transgender person's identity as a disabling condition treatable by psychotropic medication or aversive therapies.

In San Francisco, there is an expanding range of social, artistic, medical, and mental health programs oriented to address the needs of transgender individuals. The number of mental health professionals who are transgender is also increasing, as is the number of workshops on social bias issues and supportive clinical care conceived and conducted by transgender men and women. Most recently, San Francisco approved up to $50,000 per person in health benefits for transgender city workers to cover the costs of hormone treatment and sex reassignment surgery.

Scientific Study of Transgender Identity

In both children and adults, the persistence of classifying transgender identity or cross-dressing behavior as an aberrant mental disorder may be a result of negative social views rather than empirical justification. One of the critical omissions of past psychiatric clinical research has been the lack of an identified control group. Such a control group would comprise representative de-

traits, such as male and female subjects, diversity of
range of socioeconomic levels (American Psychiatric
n 1994). However, as with homosexuality, the precise
d breadth of the transgender population cannot be reliably estimated. This lack of reliable estimates is due to forces
that constrain the self-identification of transgender individuals
and the risk of negative consequences for such identification.

Psychiatric Diagnosis and Nomenclature

The fourth edition of the *Diagnostic and Statistical Manual of Mental Disorders* (DSM-IV), published by the American Psychiatric
Association in 1994, is the preeminent reference for the definition
and description of mental illnesses. Although homosexuality was
removed as a mental disorder from DSM-II (American Psychiatric Association 1968) in 1973, transgender identity remains in the
psychiatric classification under the diagnoses of transvestic fetishism (302.3), formerly transvestism; gender identity disorder
in adolescents or adults (302.85), formerly transsexualism; and
gender identity disorder in children (302.6) (see Tables 5–1 and
5–2).

Table 5–1. DSM-IV-TR diagnostic criteria for transvestic fetishism
(302.3)

A. Over a period of at least 6 months, in a heterosexual male, recurrent,
intense sexually arousing fantasies, sexual urges, or behaviors
involving cross-dressing.

B. The fantasies, sexual urges, or behaviors cause clinically significant
distress or impairment in social, occupational, or other important
areas of functioning.

Specify if:

   With gender dysphoria: if the person has persistent discomfort
   with gender role or identity

Source. Reprinted with permission from *Diagnostic and Statistical Manual of
Mental Disorders*, 4th Edition, Text Revision. Washington, DC, American Psychiatric Association, 2000. Copyright 2000, American Psychiatric Association.

Table 5–2. DSM-IV-TR diagnostic criteria for gender identity disorder

A. A strong and persistent cross-gender identification (not merely a desire for any perceived cultural advantages of being the other sex).

In children, the disturbance is manifested by four (or more) of the following:

(1) repeatedly stated desire to be, or insistence that he or she is, the other sex

(2) in boys, preference for cross-dressing or simulating female attire; in girls, insistence on wearing only stereotypical masculine clothing

(3) strong and persistent preferences for cross-sex roles in make-believe play or persistent fantasies of being the other sex

(4) intense desire to participate in the stereotypical games and pastimes of the other sex

(5) strong preferences for playmates of the other sex

In adolescents and adults, the disturbance is manifested by symptoms such as a stated desire to be the other sex, frequent passing as the other sex, desire to live or be treated as the other sex, or the conviction that he or she has the typical feelings and reactions of the other sex.

B. Persistent discomfort with his or her sex or sense of inappropriateness in the gender role of that sex.

In children, the disturbance is manifested by any of the following: in boys, assertion that his penis or testes are disgusting or will disappear or assertion that it would be better not to have a penis, or aversion toward rough-and-tumble play and rejection of male stereotypical toys, games and activities; in girls, rejection of urinating in a sitting position, assertion that she has or will grow a penis, or assertion that she does not want to grow breasts or menstruate, or marked aversion toward normative feminine clothing.

In adolescents and adults, the disturbance is manifested by symptoms such as preoccupation with getting rid of primary and secondary sex characteristics (e.g., request for hormones, surgery, or other procedures to physically alter sexual characteristics to simulate the other sex) or belief that he or she was born the wrong sex.

Table 5–2. DSM-IV-TR diagnostic criteria for gender identity disorder (*continued*)

C. The disturbance is not concurrent with a physical intersex condition.

D. The disturbance causes clinically significant distress or impairment in social, occupational, or other important areas of functioning.

Code based on current age:

    302.6   **Gender identity disorder in children**

    302.85   **Gender identity disorder in adolescents or adults**

Specify if (for sexually mature individuals):

    Sexually attracted to males

    Sexually attracted to females

    Sexually attracted to both

    Sexually attracted to neither

Source. Reprinted with permission from *Diagnostic and Statistical Manual of Mental Disorders*, 4th Edition, Text Revision. Washington, DC, American Psychiatric Association, 2000. Copyright 2000, American Psychiatric Association.

Psychiatric nomenclature pertaining to transgender identity evolved from nonmedical sources. *Transvestism*, derived from Latin roots meaning to wear the clothing of the opposite sex, has appeared in the psychiatric nomenclature since the term was coined by Magnus Hirschfeld in 1910. *Transsexualism*, named by Hirschfeld in 1923, first appeared as a diagnostic category in DSM-III (American Psychiatric Association 1980).

The term *transgender* is attributed to writer Virginia Price. Ms. Price, an American writer who was born biologically male, currently identifies and dresses full-time as a woman. She has no desire for physically transforming sex hormone administration or sex reassignment surgery. This differentiates her from transsexual women, nonoperative or preoperative. The term *transgender*, therefore, represents a broad and socially defined identification of *self*—the male or female gender identity that an individual holds as manifested psychologically or physically or according to stereotypic behavior, including the expression of male or female name, clothing, makeup, and sex role behavior.

The Intersection of Transgenderism and Homosexuality

It is important to distinguish between transgender identity and homosexual orientation.

Gender is a multivariate identity. Every person has aspects of gender defined in different ways. A person's *genetic gender* derives from the pairing of X and Y sex chromosomes on the sex-determining chromosome 46. Genetic female gender is identified by XX chromosomes on DNA analysis. Genetic males have XY genotypes. Other, less common pairings—XO, XXY, and XXX chromosomes—lead to genetic illnesses often manifested by disordered behavior. Notably, transgender persons have no genetic or chromosomal abnormalities.

For persons without a chromosomal anomaly, the appearance of female or male genital anatomy at birth determines the assignment of *anatomical* and *social* gender. Genes code for physical traits and *hormonal* gender. In a number of cases, there occurs an anatomical intersex condition, in which a person possesses internal and external genitalia of both female and male organs.

Gender identity may be experienced as a *psychological* gender that usually is established by age 4 or 5. Transgender identity must be distinguished from psychotic dysmorphogenesis by the permanence and lack of bizarre ideation (e.g., a psychotic man who believes that he is pregnant or menstruating).

Legal gender is based on a physician or midwife's visual inspection of the external genitalia of each newborn infant. The determination of gender may precede birth, when ultrasound examination provides an in utero picture of the external fetal genitalia. While the presence or absence of a penis may seem to be a reliable indicator of male biological gender, an enlarged clitoris may be mistaken for a penis at birth. Subsequently, the assigned boy may develop breasts, menstruation, or other pubertal sex characteristics that traumatically confirm the biological gender as female. As determined by the birth certificate, a legal gender assignment can be changed in many states on filing for a name or gender change. These name and gender changes are determined by individual judges on the basis of the appearance of the person in court and supporting documents, including statements from psychiatrists or other mental health professionals.

There are social influences that may define a person's *political gender.* A feminist man whose primary social group consists of lesbian women may politically identify his sexual orientation as being a "male lesbian." Another person may adopt a political gender of female or male to affiliate with and affirm a chosen gender regardless of her or his biological, anatomical, hormonal, legal, or psychological gender traits.

Gender may also be *cultural* or *spiritual* in nature. American psychiatrist Dr. Richard Green recounts the presence of "cross-gender identity" in Greek mythology, East Indian society, Roman history, Renaissance Europe, and North American Native American tribes (Green 1966). There are many historical deities whose gender was both female and male, or bigendered. The African Yoruba tribal members and their devout followers worldwide experience possession by deities or demons that are male or female, without respect for the host's biological gender. The Hijra in India are a time-honored social group of transsexual women, born as males, who undergo ritual removal of the penis to live as women and who are traditionally honored with gifts of money to ward off curses. Some North American Native American tribes identified "two-spirited people" who cross-dressed and lived out social roles, usually associated with the opposite gender (Herring 1994).

Case Vignette

Clara initially presents for psychotherapy with a chief complaint of depression and anxiety. She states that she is a devout Catholic who had been identifying as a lesbian in her relationship of 8 years with "Susan." Over the past 2 years, however, Clara had come to believe that her spiritual gender identity was truly male in nature. Despite her outward female anatomy, she had felt since age 4 or 5 that she was psychologically male. During the course of 2 years of psychodynamic individual psychotherapy and a symptom-relieving course of an antidepressant/anxiolytic medication, Clara legally changed her name to Clark and her gender from female to male by application to a state court. Now male in social gender role, Clark transformed his physical appearance through testosterone administration. He did not feel a compelling need for an anatomical sex change via phalloplasty or by bringing the hormonally enlarged clitoris into greater prominence.

Because he wished to marry according to Catholic canons, Clark requested that his psychiatrist order a chromosomal analysis. When told that the test would not be eligible for coverage by Medicaid, he agreed to pay privately for the $200 test. The test results, though disappointing to Clark, were conclusive—that Clark had a genetic female profile of XX chromosome 46, consistent with his female bodily phenotype. Undeterred by the chromosomal test results, Clark felt empowered to re-approach his parish priest. The priest consented to perform a Catholic marriage ceremony uniting Clark and Susan. The priest's decision to perform the marriage was in part supported by his understanding and acceptance of the nature of psychological gender. A statement from Clark's psychiatrist affirming his gender identity as male was considered supportive in the priest's assessment of the appropriateness of performing the marriage. Most significantly, the priest concurred with Clark's spiritual gender identification as male.

Cross-Gender Behavior and Transgender Identity in Children

Along with the inclusion of both homosexual (same-sex loving) and transgender (gender cross-living) persons in studies of sexual behavior, much clinical attention has been devoted to the gender-based behavior of children, without knowing whether cross-dressing in childhood results in heterosexual, homosexual, or transgender identity in adult life. Often for girls as well as boys, behavior or cross-dressing that is seen by parents as appropriate only to the opposite sex is a cause for the parents to call for psychiatric intervention. Despite such attempts to placate the parents by conversion (akin to antihomosexual reparative therapy) methods, DSM-IV acknowledges the futility of such treatment, noting that "by late adolescence or adulthood, about three-quarters of boys who had a childhood history of Gender Identity Disorder report a homosexual or bisexual orientation" (American Psychiatric Association 2000, p. 580; see Haldeman 1994). Since homosexuality is no longer classified as a mental disorder, psychiatric treatment that attempts to interfere with or change the sex role behavior of children is as unjustified as reparative therapy intended to change the sexual orientation of adults (Martin 1984). Reparative therapy for homosexual persons has been determined— by the American Psychological Association (1997) among others— to be disreputable.

There is an intersection between gender identity and nonstereotypical sex role behavior in children who later manifest homosexuality. DSM-IV states that up to one-quarter of boys with a history of childhood gender identity disorder may have a "concurrent Gender Identity Disorder" as adults. If the future adult homosexuality of boys with nonstereotypical sex role behavior is unaffected by psychiatric treatment, then it stands to reason that boys who come to identify as transgender persons in adulthood are apparently similarly immune to conversion or reparative therapies.

In my clinical experience with more than 100 transgender patients (in voluntary treatment for help in coping with various stressors) and with dozens of nonpatient acquaintances, there is far more distress induced by childhood histories of parental disapproval and punishment of cross-gender behavior than distress over their eventual adult gender identification.

The diminished view of cross-gender behavior of children as psychopathological parallels the evolution of psychiatry's acknowledgement that sexual orientation, per se, is not a mental disorder. Moreover, clinically significant distress can result from the negative consequences of societal pressures upon the homosexual individual. A similar biopsychosocial approach to gender diversity would no longer consider gender identity disorder ("gender dysphoria"), transsexualism, or transvestism as specific disease entities but instead would limit psychiatric treatment to recovery from the chronic societal traumas encountered by transgender individuals. Ineffective and potentially harmful psychiatric treatment efforts to suppress transgender expression in either adults or children would be considered professionally invalid as reparative therapies for homosexual persons.

Psychiatric Illness and Referral

The biopsychosocial model for psychiatric training and practice requires constant reevaluation of what constitutes a mental illness and whether specific treatments for such illnesses are necessary and beneficial and avoid harmful effects. Changes in social constructions have led the psychiatric profession to eliminate past mental diagnoses and treatments for the normative behavior of U.S. African slaves and their descendants (Lawson 1994; Pierce 1992). Within the past quarter century, social views of gay men and lesbians have changed, resulting in the psychiatric declassification of sexual orientation. Just as the concepts of psychiatric disease and remedy are no longer based on racial or sexual identity, public and professional views are changing to regard transgender children and adults as a gender minority population that has been existent and embraced in many world cultures since the earliest recorded human history. The emergence of successfully functioning transgender persons, including transgender psychiatrists and other physicians, in a progressively more tolerant and informed American society calls into question the rationale for specific diagnosis of transvestism, transsexualism, or gender identity disorder.

When there is dysphoria among transgender individuals presenting for psychiatric treatment, clinical assessment for acute and chronic trauma should be undertaken, as well as screening for treatable affective disorders and disorders most common in the general population. The prevalent and empirically validated mental disorders may include acute stress disorder, major depression, generalized anxiety disorder, social anxiety disorder, and posttraumatic stress disorder. Referrals to community support organizations, library and online Internet resources, peer support providers (Mowbray et al. 1996), and, occasionally, gender specialists (Israel and Tarver 1997) should be highly considered on the basis of the individual's stated goals.

Future psychiatric attention may shift toward the prevention of psychosocial trauma and psychiatric illness (Munoz et al. 1987). Too few efforts have been made toward studying the psychopathology of racism and racist patients (Pierce 1969), homophobia, transphobia, childhood bullying (Olweus 1991), and so forth.

Diagnostic Revision

Psychiatric perceptions of transgender persons by American psychiatrists are remarkably parallel to those for gay men and lesbians before the declassification of homosexuality as a mental disorder in 1973. The present diagnostic categories of gender identity disorder and transvestic fetishism, like drapetomania, dysaesthesia aethiopica, and homosexuality in past decades, may or may not meet current definitions of psychiatric disorder, depending on subjective assumptions about "normal" sex and gender roles and the distress of societal prejudice.

Recent revisions of the *Diagnostic and Statistical Manual of Mental Disorders* have made the categories of illness related to transgender identity increasingly ambiguous and reflect a lack of consensus within the American Psychiatric Association. The result is that a widening segment of gender-nonconforming youth and adults are potentially subject to diagnosis of psychosexual disorder, stigma, and loss of civil liberty.

Revising these diagnostic categories will not eliminate transgender stigma, but it may reduce its legitimacy, just as reform of the diagnostic classification in DSM did for homophobia in the 1970s. It is possible to define a diagnosis that specifically addresses the needs of transsexual persons requiring medical sex reassignment and provides criteria that are clearly and appropriately inclusive. It is time for the transgender community to engage the psychiatric profession in a dialogue that promotes medical and public policies that, above all, do no harm to those they are intended to help.

References

Adebimpe VR: Race, racism, and epidemiological surveys. Hosp Community Psychiatry 45:27–31, 1994

American Psychiatric Association: Diagnostic and Statistical Manual of Mental Disorders, 2nd Edition. Washington, DC, American Psychiatric Association, 1968

American Psychiatric Association: Diagnostic and Statistical Manual of Mental Disorders, 3rd Edition. Washington, DC, American Psychiatric Association, 1980

American Psychiatric Association: Diagnostic and Statistical Manual of Mental Disorders, 3rd Edition, Revised. Washington, DC, American Psychiatric Association, 1987

American Psychiatric Association: Diagnostic and Statistical Manual of Mental Disorders, 4th Edition. Washington, DC, American Psychiatric Association, 1994

American Psychiatric Association: Diagnostic and Statistical Manual of Mental Disorders, 4th Edition, Text Revision. Washington, DC, American Psychiatric Association, 2000

American Psychological Association: Resolution on appropriate therapeutic responses to sexual orientation. Adopted by the American Psychological Association Council of Representatives, August 14, 1997

Davison GC: Homosexuality: the ethical challenge. J Consult Clin Psychol 44:157–162, 1976

De Bow's Review—Southern and Western States (1851), Vol XI: New Orleans. New York, AMS Press, 1967

Green R: Transsexualism: mythological, historical, and cross-cultural aspects (Appendix C), in The Transsexual Phenomenon. Edited by Benjamin H. New York, Julian Press, 1966, pp 174–184

Haldeman D: The practice and ethics of sexual orientation conversion therapy. J Consult Clin Psychol 62:221–227, 1994

Herring RD: Native American Indian identity: a people of many peoples, in Race, Ethnicity and Self: Identity in Multicultural Perspective. Edited by Salett E, Koslow D. Washington, DC, National Multicultural Institute, 1994, pp 170–197

Israel GE, Tarver DE: Transgender Care: Recommended Guidelines, Practical Information, and Personal Accounts. Philadelphia, PA, Temple University Press, 1997, pp 14–17

Lawson WB, Hepler N, Holladay J, et al: Race as a factor in inpatient and outpatient admissions and diagnosis. Hosp Community Psychiatry 45:72–74, 1994

Martin AD: The emperor's new clothes: modern attempts to change sexual orientation, in Psychotherapy With Homosexuals. Edited by Hetrick ES, Stein TS. Washington, DC, American Psychiatric Press, 1984, pp 24–57

McLeod JD, Kessler RC: Socioeconomic status differences in vulnerability to undesirable life events. J Health Soc Behav 31:162–172, 1990

Mowbray C, Moxley D, Thrasher S, et al: Consumers as community support providers: issues created by role innovation. Community Ment Health J 32:47–67, 1996

Munoz RF, Ying Y, Arman R, et al: The San Francisco Depression Prevention Research Project: a randomized trial with medical outpatients, in Depression Prevention: Research Directions. Edited by Munoz RF. Washington, DC, Hemisphere Press, 1987, pp 199–215

Olweus D: Bullying/victim problems among school children: basic facts and effects of an intervention program, in Development and Treatment of Childhood Aggression. Edited by Rubin K, Pepler D. Hillsdale, NJ, Lawrence Erlbaum, 1991, pp 411–448

Pierce CM: Our most crucial domestic issue. Am J Psychiatry 125:1583–1584, 1969

Pierce CM: Contemporary psychiatry: racial perspectives on the past and future, in The Mosaic of Contemporary Psychiatry in Perspective. Edited by Kales A, Pierce CM, Greenblatt M. New York, Springer-Verlag, 1992, pp 99–109

Priest R: Racism and prejudice as negative impacts on African American clients in therapy. Journal of Counseling and Development 70: 213–215, 1991

Index

Page numbers printed in **boldface** *type refer to tables.*

Bisexual persons. *See also* Older
   adults; Sexual orientation
   development of sexual
      minority youth and, 12–13
   friendships and support
      networks of, 29
   use of term, 95
Board of Immigration Appeals,
   62

Case vignette, of transgender
   identity, 102–103
Cass, Vivienne, 2–3
Centers for Disease Control and
   Prevention (CDC), 6
Children. *See also* Family; Parents
   cross-gender behavior and
      transgender identity in,
      103–104
   legal proceedings involving
      custody and visitation, 41–
      48
   older sexual minority adults
      and relationships with, 28
Civil Rights Act, Title VII, 49–50
Colleges, and harassment of
   sexual minority students, 8
Coming out, and immigration or
   asylum cases, 64–65, 67.
   See also Self-disclosure
Commission on Psychotherapy
   by Psychiatrists (COPP), 87
Commitment, and development
   of sexual identity, 3
Committee for the Study of Sex
   Variants, 95–96
Concealed social stigma, aging
   and sexual orientation, 18,
   21
Confidentiality, and sexual
   conversion therapy, 86

Coping
   adolescents and development
      of sexual identity, 4
   multiple minority status, 27
Criminal law, and legal
   proceedings involving sexual
   minorities, 56–61
Crisis competence, and older
   lesbians and gay men,
   23–24
Cross-gender identity, 102, 103–
   104. *See also* Identity, sexual
Cultural gender, 102
Culture, and expression of sexual
   identity, 67. *See also* Ethnicity
Culture wars, and sexual
   conversion therapy, 81–82

Dating, and development of
   sexual minority youth, 10–12
Defense mechanisms
   development of sexual
      identity and, 2–3
Development, of sexual minority
   youth
   bisexuality and transgender-
      ism, 12–13
   ethnic minorities and, 12
   self-disclosure of sexual
      orientation and, 7–10
   sexual activity and dating
      issues, 10–12
   sexual identity and impact of
      victimization, 5–7
   sexual identity and models of,
      2–5
*Diagnostic and Statistical Manual of
   Mental Disorders* system, and
   diagnoses involving sexual
   orientation, 76, 77, 78, 98–100,
   103, 104, 106

Discrimination
  government jobs and sexual
    orientation in postwar
    years, 18–19
  impact of ageism and
    heterosexism on older
    sexual minority adults, 30–
    31
  legal proceedings on
    workplace harassment
    and, 48–56
  role of psychiatry in evolution
    of laws on, 68
  stress and older gay, lesbian,
    and bisexual persons, 25
Domestic relationship, and same-
  sex domestic violence, 61
Domestic violence, and same-sex
  relationships, 56–61
Double life, of sexual minority
  elderly, 22
Drapetomania, 94, 106
Dysaesthesia Aethiopica, 94, 106
Dysphoria, in transgender
  individuals, 105

"Ego dystonic homosexuality,"
  78
Elderly. See Older adults
Emotional distress
  immigration and asylum
    cases, 64
  workplace harassment or
    discrimination, 54, 55
Employment
  government jobs and
    discrimination in postwar
    years, 18–19
  legal proceedings on
    harassment and
    discrimination in, 48–56

Employment Non-Discrimina-
  tion Act (ENDA), 50
Equal rights, for sexual
  minorities, 37, 48
Ethics, and sexual conversion
  therapy, 72, 84–86, 87
Ethnicity. See also African
  Americans; Culture; Native
  Americans
  development of sexual
    minority youth and, 12
  multiple minorities and older
    gay, lesbian, and bisexual
    persons, 26, 27
Ex-gay movement, 79

Facts, and testimony of mental
  health professionals in legal
  proceedings, 39–40
Family, and older sexual minority
  adults, 28–30. See also
  Children; Parents; Support
  systems
Florida, and adoption of children
  by gay men or lesbians, 41–42
Ford, C., 77
Foster care, 42
Freud, Sigmund, 19–20, 73–75
Friendships, and older sexual
  minority adults, 28–29, 30.
  See also Relationships;
  Support systems

Gannet, Deborah, 96
Gay men. See also Older adults;
  Sexual orientation
  adolescents and development
    of sexual identity, 4, 5, 8,
    11–12
  friendships and support
    networks of, 29

Gay men *(continued)*
 parental relationships with
  adult children and, 28
Gay Straight Alliances, 10
Gender
 differentiation of from sexual
  orientation, 95
 as multivariate identity, 101–
  102
 social norms of, 96–97
Gender identity disorder, 93, 98,
  99–100, 103, 104, 105, 106.
  See also Identity, sexual
Genetic gender, 101
Government, employment
  discrimination and
  homosexuality in postwar
  period, 18–19. *See also* Legal
  issues and proceedings;
  States and state laws
Group therapy, for older sexual
  minority adults, 32

Harassment. *See also* Persecution;
  Sexual harassment; Verbal
  abuse; Victimization
 colleges and sexual minority
  students, 8
 legal proceedings on
  workplace, 48–56
 stress and older gay, lesbian, or
  bisexual persons, 25
Hate crimes legislation, 48,
  56–57
Health care, and sensitivity to
  gay, lesbian, bisexual, and
  transgender issues, 33
Hernandez-Montiel, Geovanni,
  62
Heterosexism, and older sexual
  minority adults, 30–31

Heterosexuality. *See also* Sexual
  orientation
 bisexual youth and self-
  identification as, 13
 dating and sexual activity of
  sexual minority youth, 11
 use of term, 95
Hetrick-Martin Institute, 7
Hirschfeld, Magnus, 100
Historical background, of current
  cohort of older adults, 18–20
Homelessness, and sexual
  minority youth, 8
Homophobia, and workplace
  harassment, 51, 55
Homosexuality. *See also* Sexual
  orientation
 culture wars and, 81–82
 religious views of, 78–81
 transgenderism and, 101–103
 use of term, 95
Homosexual panic defense, 57
Hooker, Evelyn, 77
Hormonal gender, 101
Hospitals, and sensitivity to gay,
  lesbian, bisexual, and trans-
  gender issues, 33
Hostile work environment, 48

Identity, sexual. *See also* Cross-
  gender identity; Gender
  identity disorder
 bisexual youth and
  heterosexuality, 13
 double life of older sexual
  minority adults and, 22
 impact of victimization on
  development in sexual
  minority youth, 5–7
 sexual minority youth, models
  of development, 2–5

transgender youth and self-identification issues, 13
Illness/behavior model, of homosexuality, 81–82
Immaturity, and theories of homosexuality, 71, 73–75, 78
Immigration, and legal proceedings involving sexual orientation, 61–67
Immigration Act of 1917, 61
India, and social norms of gender, 96–97, 102
Informed consent, and sexual conversion therapy, 85
International Classification of Diseases (ICD), 71
Inversion, and Freud's view of homosexuality, 73–74

Japan, study of children of mixed Asian ancestry, 21

Kinsey, Alfred, 77
Krafft-Ebing, R., 73

Legal gender, 101–102
Legal issues and proceedings. *See also* Government; States and state laws; Supreme Court
child custody and visitation and issues of sexual orientation, 41–48
criminal law and same-sex domestic violence cases, 56–61
immigration and asylum cases, 61–67
increasing number of involving lesbians and gay men, 37–38, 68

special issues for older sexual minority adults and, 34
workplace harassment and discrimination against sexual minorities, 48–56
Lesbians. *See also* Older adults; Sexual orientation
adolescents and development of sexual identity, 4
adolescents and same-sex relationships, 11, 12
ethnic minorities and children of, 12
friendships and support networks of, 29
parental relationships with adult children and, 28
same-sex domestic violence and, 60
self-disclosure of sexual orientation by adolescents and parental acceptance, 8
special issues for older adults, 34
Lorde, Audre, 27
Loss, and special issues for older gay men, 34. *See also* Bereavement

Master status, aging and sexual orientation, 18
Mattachine Society, 19
McCarthyism, and persecution of homosexuals, 18–19
Moberly, Elizabeth, 79–80
Moral fitness, and child custody and visitation disputes, 44
Motivation, and sexual orientation conversion, 84

testimony in legal proceedings by, 46–48, 52, 53–56, 63–67

Psychiatry. *See also* American Psychiatric Association; Psychiatrists
calls for moratorium on sexual conversion therapy, 87
development of views on homosexuality in postwar years, 19–20
diagnosis and nomenclature for transgenderism, 98–100
psychiatric illnesses in transgender individuals and referrals, 105
role in evolution of law or legal precedence, 68

Psychological distress, and minority stressors on older gay men and lesbians, 25

Psychological gender, 101

Psychological harm, and workplace harassment or discrimination, 54, 55

Psychotherapy, for older sexual minority adults, 33–34

Racism, 93, 94–95, 105

Rado, Sandor, 75–76

Referrals, and psychiatric illnesses in transgender individuals, 105

Refugee Act of 1980, 61–62

Relationships. *See also* Friendships; Support systems
domestic violence and same-sex, 56–61
lack of appropriate models for same-sex, 30

older adults and long-term emotionally intimate, 29–30
sexual minority youth and same-sex, 11, 12

Religion and religious views
child custody and visitation disputes involving sexual minorities and, 46
justification of slavery and, 94
sexual conversion therapy and, 78–81

Reno, Janet, 62

Reparative therapy, 79, 80–81, 104. *See also* Sexual conversion therapy

Repression, and public attitudes toward sexual orientation in postwar years, 18–20

Resilience, and psychological research on aging sexual minorities, 26

Responses, to self-disclosure of sexual orientation by adolescents, 7–8

Retirement, of older adults in sexual minority communities, 20

Role models
for multiple minorities, 27
for same-sex relationships, 30

Safe Schools Coalition of Washington, 6

SAGE (Senior Action in a Gay Environment), 26

Same-sex sexual harassment, 49

San Francisco, and ordinance prohibiting discrimination based on gender identity, 97

"Second parent adoption," 42

States and state laws. *See also* Government; Legal issues and proceedings
  adoption by gay or lesbian parents and, 41–42
  child custody or visitation disputes involving sexual minorities, 42–43, 44, 45
  workplace harassment based on sexual orientation and, 50
Stigma, and older adults in gay, lesbian, bisexual, and transgender communities, 18, 21–26
Stonewall Inn bar (New York City), police raid in 1969, 20
Stress
  impact of on older lesbians and gay men, 23, 24–26, 32
  legal proceedings on workplace harassment or discrimination and, 55–56
Suicide and suicidal ideation, prevalence of in older gay, lesbian, or bisexual persons, 24
Support systems. *See also* Family; Friendships; Relationships; Social services
  development of sexual minority youth and, 10
  for older gay, lesbian, and bisexual persons, 24, 28–29
Supreme Court, and lesbian or gay publications, 19. *See also* Legal issues and proceedings
Survivors, and research studies on older gay men and lesbians, 22

Tenorio, Marcelo, 62
Toboso-Alfonso, Fidel Armando, 62
Transgender individuals. *See also* Older adults; Sexual orientation
  children and cross-gender behavior, 103–104
  development of sexual minority youth and, 12–13
  differentiation of gender from sexual orientation, 95
  history of studies on, 95–96
  homosexuality and, 101–103
  psychiatric diagnosis and nomenclature, 98–100
  psychiatric illness and referral, 105
  reevaluation and depathologizing of, 93
  scientific study of identity and, 97–98
  social norms of gender and, 96–97
  special issues of older persons and, 32
Transsexualism, 100, 104, 105
Transvestic fetishism, 98, 106
Transvestism, 100, 104, 105

Ulrichs, Karl, 72, 74
University of Florida, 19
Unwelcomed behaviors, and sexual harassment, 53–54

Verbal abuse, of older gay, lesbian, or bisexual persons, 25. *See also* Harassment

Victimization. *See also* Harassment
  development of sexual identity in adolescents and, 5–7
  stress and older gay, lesbian, or bisexual persons, 24, 25–26
Violent behaviors, and same-sex domestic violence, 59–60

Wall Street Journal, 82
White, Mel, 83–84

Women's rights movement, 20, 59
Workplace harassment, and legal proceedings, 48–56

Yale University, 8
Yoruba (Africa), and gender as multivariate identity, 102
Youth. *See* Adolescents
Youth Risk Behavior Survey (YRBS), 6